Living Cancer

Stories of an
Oncologist, Father, Survivor

MICHAEL WEINER, MD

LIVING CANCER: STORIES OF AN ONCOLOGIST, FATHER, SURVIVOR

1405 SW 6th Avenue • Ocala, Florida 34471 • Phone 352-622-1825 • Fax 352-622-1875
Website: www.atlantic-pub.com • Email: sales@atlantic-pub.com
SAN Number: 268-1250

Library of Congress Control Number: 2020908186

Printed in the United States

PROJECT MANAGER: Jessie Ranew
INTERIOR LAYOUT AND JACKET DESIGN: Nicole Sturk

Table of Contents

Foreword

I knew that something was wrong when my daughter, Leilah, five, fell asleep in my arms at our Passover dinner. She was usually a bundle of non-stop energy but for the past several days she had been tired and pale. Increasingly tired and pale. We were on vacation at a ski resort in Snowbird, Utah, and usually she loved to take the kid's ski lessons, but not on this trip. I was already worried about her and had taken her to the clinic the day we arrived. The doctor had examined her and told me with assurance—"she just has a little bug." But now, I decided that we would go back first thing the next morning.

That would be the beginning of an over two-year journey, that was an emotional rollercoaster of fear and hope. To his credit, the clinic doctor decided to do a chest x-ray of Leilah, suspecting that she might have pneumonia even though she was only running a low-grade fever. "Come take a look at this," he called me over to see the x-ray a few minutes later. "Does Leilah have a heart abnormality? It looks like her heart is enlarged."

"No," I gulped, immediately worried. The doctor and I dialed my pediatrician right away. When he came on the phone, he tried to calm me down, assuring me that the x-ray was probably low-quality, and that Leilah most likely had an infection of some type. But my "mom instincts" were on full alert. Eight years earlier, my older daughter, Sofia, had had to have emergency surgery for what turned out to be a brain tumor, when she had just turned three. It had been me who just 'knew' she had a tumor when she told me her head hurt just a few days before that. My husband and our pediatrician at the time thought I was nuts when I had insisted on taking Sofia to the local hospital at 6 in the morning after her head hurt so much that it woke her up.

Thankfully, after two 12-hour surgeries, a week apart, the tumor was successfully removed and wasn't malignant. We had been very, very lucky once. Now, I wasn't taking any chances with my younger daughter's health. My husband didn't object when I told him we needed to go home that day. We packed up our three other children hurriedly and caught a flight home to New York City that afternoon.

Our anxieties only increased when we got back and it took two days for our insurance company to approve a CT scan for Leilah, as she grew increasingly weak. But, when our pediatrician got the results, he immediately flew into action and came back with a plan. "I've contacted the Children's Hospital at Columbia Presbyterian on New York City's Upper West Side," he said. "You have an appointment there tomorrow at 10:30 a.m. with Leilah." He didn't know if Leilah had a lymphoma or a leukemia, but she did have what appeared to be cancer cells all around the outside lining around her heart (explaining why her heart looked enlarged on the x-ray). There were masses on her liver and kidneys and on her lymph nodes. We were devastated. Not again. The life of another one of our precious babies was threatened. Poor, sweet Leilah.

We were terrified.

My husband and I could barely sleep that night, holding Leilah between us. We feared Leilah wouldn't have a chance. When Michael and I grew up in the 1960s and early 1970s, leukemia was a disease that was considered a death sentence. Parents prayed that their children would not be struck down by the mysterious bleeding disease.

Now, we knew that great progress had been made in treating leukemia, but we were too afraid to start Googling for more information on survival rates that night. We didn't know yet, what Leilah's diagnosis would be and we knew we had to try to keep up our strength and hope. Whatever would happen the next day or in the coming weeks, we knew it would be an emotional marathon.

At exactly 10:30 a.m. we arrived at the check-in desk of the children's pavilion at Columbia Presbyterian Hospital. Michael had Leilah in his arms—she was too tired to walk. We assumed that we would be waiting a while for Dr. Michael Weiner—the name our pediatrician had given us.

But, barely a few moments had passed—we hadn't even had time to sit down—when an energetic man came around the corner and walked right over to us to say hello. "I'm Dr. Michael Weiner, the director of pediatric oncology here. Is this Leilah? Hi, sweetie." He immediately took a quick look at Leilah's face. She could barely lift her little head.

"Here's what I'm going to tell you," he stared right at us. "I'm going to save your daughter."

And he did. She had Acute Lymphoblastic Leukemia (ALL). It took two long years of intense chemotherapy and radiation treatments, stints of staying in the hospital, urgent trips back there, and a strict adherence to the required treatment's protocol, but thank God, Leilah made it. Today, Leilah is a beautiful, healthy 23-year-old young woman.

I truly don't believe that she would be here today without Dr. Weiner's expertise, passion, and determination. He had built a dedicated and highly knowledgeable pediatric oncology team at Columbia Presbyterian. Leilah, as it turned out, had a rarer and more aggressive form of ALL than the typical case and it was called T-cell ALL. It had a lower survival rate than the more common B-cell ALL. But, fortunately the hospital had a new, more aggressive, and experimental protocol for Leilah's cancer—it was only offered at a couple of hospitals across the country. Thank goodness we were with Dr. Weiner and his team. The treatment was successful and from what I understand, is now the standard for T-cell ALL, with a much-improved survival rate.

But, as you will learn from the real life and death stories that Dr. Weiner relates in this book, *Living Cancer: Stories of an Oncologist, Father, Survivor,* he applies the same warmth and deep commitment and compassion to all the children and teenagers he has treated. He doesn't fear becoming emotionally involved with his patients. They are never just a "case" to him, to be clinically treated and studied.

Along with working with his team to determine the best possible and up to date treatments for even the most difficult and acute cases of cancer, he also takes late night phone calls from worried parents, always with a calm reassurance: I know. I made these calls.

I can confirm to you that when you read about the children, young people, and parents that he has written about on these pages, their experiences and his all ring true, and all feel very personal. My husband, Michael, and I couldn't be more grateful to Dr. Weiner, Dr. Kara Kelly, and the dedicated team that treated Leilah.

If you are a parent with a child battling cancer, this book should give you hope. There are doctors like Dr. Weiner, armed with knowledge, science, and dedication who will fight with everything in their arsenal to save your child.

And today, they often win.

Bonnie Fuller
Editor-in-Chief of Hollywood Life
Mother of Four

Preface

Cancer is ubiquitous; its reach inescapable. It touches every family in America, making its insidious presence known when least expected, often without warning. Cancer does not discriminate; regardless of economic status, race, gender, or geographic location, we are all susceptible to its ravages. When cancer knocks, one has little choice but to open the door and let it in.

As a species, we have built civilizations, waged wars, and created religion in an attempt to grapple with our own mortality and shared fear of death. Childhood cancer is especially devastating. Human predisposition and instincts throughout the animal kingdom dictate that we protect the young. To see a child ill with any disease from the most banal ear infection to serious, acute, and chronic conditions is devastating to parents. When a child, your child, is diagnosed with cancer it is deeply unsettling, wrenching—the world spins out of control. Parents desperately attempt to shield and safeguard their child but find their efforts thwarted as they lose control to the disease and the very treatment intended to ameliorate the cancer.

Childhood and adolescent cancer is not common. In the United States, there are only 15,000 newly diagnosed cases of childhood cancer each year—a small number compared to the 1.7 million newly diagnosed adults. A pediatrician in a robust practice might see one or two cases diagnosed in his professional career; a town or school system, the same. When it does occur, childhood cancer is like a hurricane, destroying everything in its path, leaving families alone, gutted, and forced to rebuild their lives.

As a pediatric oncologist for more than 40 years, I have worked with children and parents who have been touched by these catastrophic diseases. Despite the fact that I have been practicing for so many years and have cared for thousands of patients and families, I remember each. The stories I have chosen to share with the reader within this book, however, are particularly memorable because they are the cases in which I became unusually close with either the patient, their family, or the circumstances regarding my relationship with them.

I have had the great honor and pleasure of treating some truly remarkable children, like Bill Oliver, a young man whose future as an exceptional long-distance runner was abruptly halted his senior year of high school by a rare carcinoma. I spent countless hours talking with Bill's mother, Anne, as her son endured an unimaginable year of chemotherapy, radiation, and surgery. The insight gleaned from our discussion was enlightening on so many levels; I learned much from Anne. However, our conversations are not exact, or precise, but rather my recollection of the dialogue.

I often think about Tania Small, a young girl raised in Brooklyn by a single mother, whose previous heart transplant led her to develop an unusual type of acute leukemia.

Spending time with these children and their families during some of the most painful and terrifying moments of their lives, I found myself in a unique position, serving primarily as doctor but also, as was the case with the family of Bill Oliver, as confidant; or as was the case with Tania Small, as surrogate parent. It is a strange role to play, and while I attempted to lend my own experience, guidance, and expertise to new and returning patients, on a personal level, the pain and upset never truly subsided.

The experiences I had with my patients were further informed by my personal experiences with cancer. My daughter, Lauren, was diagnosed with thyroid cancer at the age of 24, and I myself was diagnosed and treated for a type of non-Hodgkin's lymphoma as an adult. I have experienced cancer from all sides of the table, as a doctor, as a parent, and as a patient—truly a

360-degree view. The result has been a sometimes-uncomfortable intimacy with this terrible disease.

Although each patient is distinct, their stories are interconnected. Each narrative reflects my experiences and observations, and for that reason, the book often becomes a stream of consciousness—a mosaic of cancer journeys, all of which lead toward the same essential human truths. Even though my personal cancer experience and that of my daughter, Lauren, may appear less intense than the reflections of my patients, it does not diminish—not one iota—the terrifying fact that cancer is cancer and people die from these diseases.

I know that my experiences, though vast, are not unique. Books and stories about cancer seem as abundant as the disease itself, though few touch the raw emotion of the patients and families, allowing the reader to reflect upon the despair, courage, pain, suffering, and at times, triumph of this horrific illness.

What I hope to offer in this book is a collection of true and personal tales of hope, bravery, pain, survival, and resilience in the face of the unimaginable. So many of us are suffering in silence, whether at the hands of a disease, an oppressive situation, or our own internal setbacks. What I've come to understand during my many years working closely with this disease and its repercussions is that pain and suffering are better dealt with when they are expressed and shared. In hearing stories, not only of hardship, but of joy, love, humor, and most of all, true, lived experience, we as human beings are able to learn empathy and better support one another. It is my hope that these stories will empower the reader to learn, to understand, and to enrich their existence.

As a structuring technique, I employ the routine of "rounds," moving with my team of medical students, residents, fellows, and nurses from room to room on the pediatric oncology inpatient unit to check on patients. As a team we discuss each case and learn something new each and every day. In each room is a different patient, with each patient comes a unique story.

Through each of these patients and their stories, I was able to learn about myself—my own ability to give and receive care, and the ways in which my own life experiences are both a help and a hindrance to my ability to do my job. In my own story, and the story of my daughter Lauren, I more deeply examine these ideas, looking at how my past behaviors—good, bad, and ugly—have come to determine my current relationships and career. Of course, this emotional excavation can at times be deeply painful, and I hope that that pain similarly resonates on the page. Perhaps my biggest takeaway from my experiences and from the writing of these stories has been that we, as people, are constantly navigating the parameters of pain, just as we are navigating those of love. Sharing our experiences, especially the challenges, gives us strength to grow and develop.

Any patient will tell you that proximity to death brings with it proximity to life. I hope that this book will lead readers toward a more intense awareness of their living self—their truest self.

You are never more alive than when you are almost dead.

Living Cancer: Stories of an Oncologist, Parent, Survivor is a book about cancer and the people who live it. Throughout the book, the reader will come to know some of the many facets of this insidious disease as we examine the personal stories of seven former patients, as well as my daughter Lauren's cancer story and my own. The reader will be in the room with me, my team, and my patients, witnessing first-hand the conversations, emotions, and complexities of care of each distinct case.

The reader will be introduced to patients whose lives were tragically lost, despite aggressive treatment; and patients for whom treatment worked, wholly or partially. We will encounter patients suffering unusual malignancies, infection, lung failure, and anaphylactic reactions; patients received aggressive chemotherapy, blood transfusions, and experimental treatment. Though there are differences in the diagnosis, treatment, and, of course, the patients themselves and their families, we will come to see that there are also overwhelming similarities. Fundamentally driven toward life, the struggle to survive and to love is keenly felt in each patient.

Regardless of disease outcome, cancer can teach us lessons applicable to myriad life situations; it alters and empowers all who come in contact with it. These lessons become more immediately emotional and accessible when I discuss my daughter's and my own cancer diagnosis. These memories are deeply personal, and while there are parallels to be drawn, and certainly my experience dealing with cancer patients informed this experience, nothing could have prepared me. Through my daughter, I came to understand first-hand what the parents of Hank Held or Harris Schulman had been dealing with. The reality and abject fear as a parent is, of course, indescribable, but within these chapters I attempt to impart my experience as vividly as words allow.

The reader will meet Mark Alan Nieman, a young man who asked his parents, "If only I had leukemia, I would be cured, right Mom?" He pleaded with his parents, Madeline and Frank, "You're smart—please do something!" The Niemans have changed the world for so many.

This book offers a unique look at how care-making decisions are made by doctors. These decisions are often made in a manner than may seem almost as cavalier as tossing a coin; only in the case of cancer, an incorrect guess may be catastrophic. Endless thought, deliberation, study, and consideration go into these decisions, but ultimately, it is not an exact science. Much as I wish it were otherwise, there are many situations in which the outcome is a mystery.

Throughout the book, I examine the mechanics and bureaucracies of treating cancer within a hospital. In discussing the trajectory of my career and the many medical professionals I've come in contact with, I more closely examine the corporate nature of large academic medical centers, and specifically, the ways in which their size and structure affect process. I speak candidly about some of the challenges I've encountered professionally—both interpersonally with other doctors and administrators, and structurally.

The reflections contained within the pages of *Living Cancer: Stories of an Oncologist, Father, Survivor*, including patients, families, my daughter and my own are real; however, temporally some stories are recollections from decades ago, thus the precise dialogue, although based on factual situations may out of necessity be fictitious. Additionally, dialogue exists that is gleaned not from personal interactions, but ascertained by taking a careful past medical history from the patient and parent, and by a review of the patient's electronic medical record; such conversations, although based on real situations and fact, are fabricated. On rare occasions, in order to preserve the flow of the story, I have inserted situations and dialogue that are contrived.

In an effort to protect privacy, every name—patient, parent, colleague, friend, and family member—except my own has been changed.

About the Author

For over four decades, Dr. Michael Weiner has worked as a pediatric oncologist alongside some of the brightest doctors in the world in some of our nation's top medical facilities. His hard work has been recognized and rewarded through great professional success, including serving as head of Pediatric Oncology at Columbia Presbyterian for many years, and re-building the Division of Pediatric Oncology at the former Babies Hospital into one of the most prominent divisions in the country. He has made major contributions in the diagnosis and treatment of patients with lymphoma, specifically Hodgkin's lymphoma, and has been nationally recognized as a leader in the field.

Despite his professional accomplishments, Dr. Weiner is most proud of the work he's done with Hope & Heroes. Hope & Heroes Children's Cancer Fund is a 501(c)(3) grassroots charitable organization he founded 22 years ago to support patients and families, education, special programs, and research at Columbia University Irving Medical Center. Since its inception, the organization has raised $100 million for those in need.

TANIA SMALL

The Almost Miracle

We completed team rounds on Tower 5, and I went to the pediatric intensive care unit on 11 Central alone. I entered room 1105 and approached the bed.

"I trusted you. You lied to me. You let me down."

These were the last words spoken to me by Tania Small. She died peacefully shortly thereafter.

Tania touched me as few others have. We shared a special bond; I was not only her doctor, I was her friend, and, in some ways, a surrogate parent, as well.

Tania had a tragic life; illness and social upheaval were her world. She was raised by her single mother, Shaneka Brown, in Section Eight Housing projects in Canarsie, Brooklyn. She never knew her father, which was probably a blessing. The housing projects rise astride the Belt Parkway. They are a foreboding sight from the road and have a reputation for gangs, drugs, and violence. Rat-infested buildings, broken elevators, no hot water to shower, nor heat during the winter, and the nightly sound of gunshots were the norm for Tania. She grew up with a revolving door of strange men sleeping with her mother.

Her mother worked at the Belvedere Nursing Home in Coney Island as a nurse's aide. She despised the work, feeding and cleaning urine and feces from the elderly, debilitated Jewish people whose children didn't want them around anymore, but it helped pay the rent and bills. Out of necessity, and without alternatives, Tania spent much time alone in the three-room apartment on the ninth floor of Building 4, 11-04 Mayor Dinkins Way.

One afternoon while in the fourth grade at Public School 141, she contracted a bad cold and cough; her temperature rose to 103 degrees. Shivering and nauseated she called her mother at work.

"Mom, I don't feel good. I have a fever, and I'm gonna throw up."

"Try to drink some water and get in bed. I can't leave work until 6, and I have a few stops to make before I can get home."

Crying, Tania said, "But I need you. I don't feel good. I'm sick."

"Stop crying. I'll be home when I can."

Shaneka arrived home at 9 p.m. She and a co-worker had a quick dinner at a nearby Burger King and went shopping for bargains at the Target Superstore in the Gateway Center just off the Belt Parkway. When she unlocked the door and entered the sparsely furnished apartment Tania was asleep in bed.

Tania was asleep in bed. Her room was small and dark. It had a single bed, dresser, chair, and a desk underneath a north-facing window that was so covered with dirt and soot that hardly any ambient light shone through. There was a small multi-colored area rug covering part of the faux composite-wood floor and two posters, one of Beyoncé and the other of Jennifer Lopez.

Shaneka was alone in her bedroom when Tania awoke at 11:30 that night.

"Mom, I can't breathe."

"What do you mean you can't breathe? What are you talking about?"

Fortunately, her mother was awake and alert enough to notice that her daughter was, in fact, having difficulty breathing. Shaneka tried to comfort her but recognized that something was terribly wrong. She dialed 911 on her cell phone.

"My daughter can't breathe. Hurry up! We need an ambulance," she said to the dispatcher. "Hurry."

When the fire department ambulance arrived 30 minutes later, Tania was beginning to turn blue. The Emergency Medical Technicians (EMTs) immediately placed her on a stretcher, attached EKG leads to monitor her heart rate, and administered oxygen through a face mask attached to a portable tank. They started an IV in her left arm for fluid hydration, gave her a small dose of Ativan to relax her, and told Shaneka to get the elevator, which was thankfully working. The oxygen and Ativan worked immediately, and Tania stabilized. They transported her to the waiting ambulance in the building courtyard where a crowd of curious onlookers had gathered to see what was happening.

The police officers who arrived on the scene shouted, "Step back. Hey you! I'm talking to you! Move back—now!"

The ambulance carrying Tania and Shaneka sped through the streets with sirens blasting and lights flashing. It took 15 minutes to reach Brookdale Hospital. The streets were alive and crowded at 1:30 a.m.—they are always crowded; cars choked the roadways.

The emergency room at Brookdale is like all busy city hospitals: crowded with humanity, some truly sick and others with colds and stomach viruses who utilize hospital emergency departments as primary care givers. The area is massive; it occupies virtually the entire first floor wing of the hospital. With doctors, nurses, assistants, technicians, hospital security guards, police officers, patients, and family members everywhere, the walls were bursting at the seams.

The ambulance arrived at the patient receiving dock where they wheeled Tania into an acute care bed in the pediatric area that was reserved for such cases. The nurses and the EMTs transferred her from the stretcher to a hospital bed. They hooked her up to monitoring devices and flushed her IV with a small dose of heparin to prevent clots from forming. Her vital signs were markedly abnormal: heart rate 125; respiratory rate 54; temperature 104. A portable chest x-ray taken at the bedside revealed fluid in her lungs and an enlarged heart. The EKG showed that her heart was weakened and not pumping blood effectively. This was no ordinary cold.

The pediatric emergency room physician at Brookdale told Shaneka Brown that she suspected there might be a problem with Tania's heart and she wanted to transfer her to Columbia, New York Presbyterian.

"What for? What's the problem? You're crazy! There's nothing wrong with my daughter's heart. She has a bad cold. I can't go to the city; I got work in 5 hours."

"Mrs. Brown, my name is Dr. Daggert."

"Don't call me Mrs. Brown. It's Miss. Brown."

"Okay, Miss Brown, let me make this as simple as I can. Your daughter is in serious trouble, her heart is failing. She needs immediate medical attention from pediatric cardiologists, and the best doctors are at Columbia University Medical Center in Upper Manhattan. We can stabilize Tania here temporarily, but we are not equipped to deal with her medical problems at Brookdale. Frankly, Miss Brown, your daughter could die if she doesn't get immediate expert medical attention and care."

"You're crazy," Shaneka insisted. "She has a bad cold. Let me speak to the doctor in charge."

Tania was resting comfortably. The doctors gave her digoxin to support her cardiac function and a light sedative to let her rest. The oxygen helped as well—her respiratory rate slowed to a normal range and her oxygen saturation returned to the low 90s. She was stable for now. Shaneka and Dr. Daggert found a small, empty consultation room adjacent to the pediatric area of the emergency room. Dr. Strong, an older man in his 50s, joined them. The room was sparsely furnished with four folding chairs and was the size of a bathroom with drab gray walls. Dr. Strong was of average size, build, and appearance, nothing notable or memorable about him. He spoke softly, slowly, and authoritatively.

"Ms. Brown," he said. "Tania is in the early stages of heart failure. Her heart is not working effectively. Her organs and brain could become oxygen starved. Fluid is accumulating in her lungs. She is in trouble and must be transferred to a hospital that specializes in children with heart disease."

"How could this happen? She was fine when she left for school this morning. She called me and said she had a cold."

"Yes, I am certain this started as a cold," said Dr. Strong. "But the virus that caused the cold and fever has attacked her heart. This is called an acute infectious cardiomyopathy. She needs skilled medical care. She needs to be transferred to Columbia; that is one of the best places in the country for children with heart problems. We need to transport her immediately."

"Are you telling me my daughter could die?"

"Yes. We are telling you that Tania is very sick, and we don't have the capabilities to care for her at Brookdale."

"Fuck this. I gotta get to work. I can't miss another day, or I'll get fired."

"Look, we have no choice here. Go to Columbia, and if we're wrong, at least you will know for sure. We can have one of the social workers call your work and explain the situation to them. That should help. Is there anyone else you can call? Do you have a car?"

"Only my mother, and she's sick, too—asthma and diabetes."

"What about her father?"

"That asshole is nowhere to be found. I haven't seen him in years. We were together when I was a teenager; he knocked me up, and I never saw him again. I doubt he even knows he has a daughter. Forget about him."

Dr. Strong said, "Look I am sorry, really sorry about your situation, but right now we have a potentially really sick girl on our hands, and we've got to get her to Columbia. Dr. Daggert is speaking to the doctors in their cardiac intensive care unit, and they will accept her tonight. We must move quickly. We need your permission to proceed, and they also want to speak with you directly. They need information about your insurance or Medicaid."

"Okay, okay," Shaneka acquiesced. "Where do I sign?"

"You're doing the right thing. Thanks. We need to tell Tania that she is going to be transferred to another hospital in New York City."

"Can you tell her?"

Shaneka calmed down and was less confrontational; she realized and understood what Drs. Daggert and Strong told her to be true. She had no choice but to transfer her daughter to the city. The small dose of Xanax that Dr. Daggert gave her also helped her relax.

"Tania, my name is Dr. Strong, and your mom and I were just talking. We need to send you to another hospital in New York City. Your cold has caused a weakness in your heart and the doctors in New York specialize in this problem. There's an ambulance on the way to take you there right now. Do you have any questions?"

Tania was too tired to speak, not only from the lateness of the hour, but also from the sedative medications she'd been administered. She was also only 10 years old and was honestly not able to process what Dr. Strong had told her. She felt sick and frightened.

She raised her head and softly asked, "I'm gonna be okay, right? Where is my mother?"

"Yes, you'll be fine. The doctors and the hospital in New York are really excellent and they will take good care of you—promise."

The transport ambulance from New York Presbyterian arrived at Brookdale at around 5 a.m. The EMTs from NYP moved Tania's stretcher onto the medical bus and helped Shaneka climb aboard as well. Traffic was light this time of morning before the onslaught of rush hour, and the ambulance crossed the East River from Brooklyn into Manhattan easily, moving quickly through the Brooklyn Battery Tunnel before heading north on FDR to the Harlem River Drive and exiting at 178th Street. The hospital was only a few blocks away on the corner of Broadway and 165th Street. The ambulance backed into the patient receiving bay, and the techs quickly wheeled Tania through the basement maze of the children's hospital until they reached the tower elevators and pressed "9" for the cardiac intensive care unit. As the elevator doors opened into the unit, the charge nurse directed them to Tower Room 905.

Tania was comfortable in her new surroundings. Room 905 was large, the bed was comfortable, and there was sofa bed for Shaneka. Beth Schultz, Tania's assigned nurse, was friendly, competent, and encouraging. She told Tania, as she connected the heart monitor and started a new intravenous line, that she was glad she was there and that the heart doctors were really excellent. She promised Tania that she would be fine. Tania did not answer but smiled shyly while Shaneka reclined on the sofa bed and closed her eyes. They were both exhausted, neither mother nor daughter had had any real sleep in the last two days.

Dr. Elizabeth Longo entered Tania's ICU room a few minutes after 9 a.m. Elizabeth is the director of the heart failure program; we have known one another for nearly 40 years. Her career has paralleled significant advances in heart failure management at Columbia, including her participation in the first successful heart transplant in a child more than 30 years ago. Elizabeth's expertise and wealth of knowledge make her a truly first-rate doctor, but it is her kindness, compassion, and empathy that make her extraordinary. She is rightfully considered one of the preeminent physicians at Columbia.

After a careful examination and testing, Elizabeth told Tania and her mother that her cold virus had mysteriously affected and weakened her heart. She told them that over the course of the next few days, there would be many tests, blood work, genetic testing, EKGs, ECHO cardiograms, CT scans, and an MRI of Tania's heart. Elizabeth indicated that the doctors and nurses needed to learn as much about Tania as possible and, in the meantime, told them that Tania would receive medications that would make her heart work more efficiently and effectively.

Shaneka asked Dr. Longo two questions. "Will Tania be all right?" was the first. The second, "Do I need to stay at the hospital? I have to get to work."

Elizabeth was taken aback by Miss Brown's cavalier tone but said, "We will need you to sign consent forms for tests and procedures now, before you leave. To be certain we can reach you, we'll need your cell phone number. When will you return to the hospital?"

"I will be back after work. I work at a nursing home in Coney Island; it's a long subway ride to Upper Manhattan, but I will try to be back tonight. I'll call my mother and see if she can stay with Tania."

To no one's surprise, Tania spent the next few days alone in the cardiac ICU. She spoke with her mother several times a day; Shaneka always answered her cell phone when her daughter called. The tests revealed that Tania had a condition known as a cardiomyopathy. The viral infection triggered an autoimmune response whereby her heart was recognized as foreign and her own antibodies attacked her heart muscle. The tests all indicated that Tania was experiencing significant heart failure. Dr. Longo prescribed high dosages of steroids as well as heart medicines. She called Miss Brown's cell phone and told her that the next week would be vital in determining whether Tania would respond to treatment. If not, she might need a heart transplant.

"What are you talking about? You must be crazy! Heart transplant? My daughter doesn't need a heart transplant. Can't you make her better? When is she gonna come home?"

"Ms. Brown, we're all doing everything we can for Tania, but her heart function is getting worse by the day. She's receiving maximum dosages of the medicines needed to improve her heart function, but nothing seems to be working. We need you at the hospital today; we want to try an experimental therapy called plasmapheresis. I have also spoken to Dr. Castille, chief of heart surgery, about putting Tania on the heart transplant list to identify a potential donor. We need you. Your daughter needs you."

Dr. Longo told Miss Brown that an ECHO is a simple test to measure heart function, and that Tania had been assessed serially, every other day. When admitted 10 days prior, her ejection fraction was 41—low but acceptable.

"Today, despite all that we are doing, it is 24—a very low level that is consistent with significant heart failure. We want to try a plasmapheresis to remove the antibody in her blood that is attacking her heart. No guarantees, but it may work. The doctors from the blood bank do the procedure, and they have time this afternoon. We need you to be here to sign the consent and to be with your daughter."

"Okay, I'll be there. When will it start, and how long does it take?"

"I'll call them now. It takes about two hours. It's quite safe, but I'll let the doctors performing the test explain it to you."

The plasmapheresis began at 2 p.m. The purpose was to remove from her blood the antibodies that were attacking her heart and causing it to fail. She tolerated the procedure well, but it failed to halt the downward spiral of heart failure. Her ejection fraction reached 18. She was critical and placed at the top of the list of patients in need of a heart transplant.

Two nights later, Tania had her heart. The New York State Organ Donation team identified an organ from a young man who had been killed in an auto accident in Albany, New York. The family consented to allow their deceased son's organs to be used to save the lives of four patients waiting for transplanted hearts, livers, lungs, and kidneys. The organs were surgically removed at Albany Medical Center, placed on ice, and transported via helicopter to several hospitals around the state. Tania's new heart arrived at midnight.

Dr. Castille and his team performed the procedure flawlessly; they removed the diseased heart and replaced it with the new, stronger organ by attaching it to the aorta, pulmonary arteries, and vena cava; dramatic for certain, but not technically difficult for the skilled surgeons led by Sergio Castille.

The next day, Tania's new heart worked like a charm. Her ejection fraction registered above 50—normal. She continued on the high dosages of steroids and began a new medicine, tacrolimus, to prevent rejection. She was discharged from the hospital a week later and returned to school three months later. Drs. Castille and Longo were very pleased with Tania's progress; they followed her closely with blood work, EKGs, ECHOs, and periodic cardiac biopsies to ascertain signs of organ failure or rejection, but there were none. The tacrolimus kept her immune system in check and prevented her body's lymphocytes from attacking her new heart.

The summer of 2018 was different.

Tania was getting ready to enter her senior year at Canarsie High School. She was thinking about college and envisioning a career in nursing. Her dream school was the nursing program at Hunter College. However, during a routine check-up with Dr. Longo, Tania's blood work revealed an abnormal white blood cell count. Elizabeth contacted me and asked my opinion, and we decided that I would see Tania that afternoon in consultation.

Tania and Miss Brown walked to my office on Irving-7 from the cardiology offices on the second floor of the north building of the children's hospital. I greeted them at the reception desk, introduced myself, and led them to one of the exam rooms. Mother and daughter resembled one another in appearance and both dressed in tee shirts, jeans with holes in the knees, and sandals.

"Dr. Longo called and asked me to review your blood work from this morning. I have read your history and know of your heart transplant seven years ago. I understand you have been quite well, is that correct?"

"Yes. I feel well; no problems. Is there something wrong with my blood?"

I told Tania and Miss Brown that her white blood cell count was low. The other blood cells, hemoglobin, and platelets were normal. We weren't certain of the significance. I asked if she had been sick with any cold or stomach virus recently, and she said that she had not. I asked Tania if we could draw another blood test, a peripheral flow, a screening test, to determine if any abnormal cells existed in her blood.

"Of course. When will we know the result?"

"Tomorrow."

Tania had leukemia.

Throughout my career I have had a golden rule: *Do not give bad news to patients and families by phone, by instant messaging, or email. Always, always in person.*

For many patients, their families, and their loved ones, the day that they receive bad news, whether an initial diagnosis or a malignant test result, will be the worst day of their lives. Of course, this is especially true when it comes to childhood cancer.

Bad news necessitates a complete restructuring of daily life and its many routines, not only for the patient but for everyone in their orbit. It may lead to job loss, financial hardship, and strained relationships in addition to the obvious and terrifying reality of having to face mortality. The effects of illness manifest in myriad ways, but it is always terrible, and for that reason, news must be delivered in person. As their doctor, I owe it to my patients and their families to be fully present. I owe it to them to look them in the eye and, to the best of my ability, provide comfort and reassurance.

In the case of Tania Small, I had no other option but to deliver the news over the phone. Tania and her mother had been expecting results from her blood tests for days, and they had already let me know that they were not going to be able to return to the hospital.

Reluctantly, I dialed Miss Brown's cell phone. She answered my call immediately. With trepidation, I gave her the bad news that Tania had abnormal blast cells in her blood, that we suspected leukemia, and that we'd need to do a bone marrow test to confirm our suspicion. Although a diagnosis of leukemia was clear, an assessment of the bone marrow would provide much needed information regarding the type of leukemia, cytogenetics, and a molecular profile; it had to be done. I told her the bone marrow test was scheduled for the next day in the ENDO procedure room.

"It takes only a few minutes."

I did the bone marrow aspirate and biopsy; Tania tolerated it well. She was stable, and her complete blood count levels did not put her at any risk of infection, bleeding, or strain on her heart. I sent her home with an appointment to return the following Monday. I spoke with Ali Mahesh, one of the hematopathologists, about the marrow findings, and he was perplexed. The tools in his toolbox are significant and cutting edge, but he indicated that Tania's marrow did not have clearly delineated lineage. Ninety-eight percent of child and adolescent leukemias are derived from lymphoid or myeloid precursors, and treatment is designed accordingly. Occasionally, the leukemia possesses markers for both lymphoid and myeloid, or they lack either marker. These unusual cases are referred to as ambiguous or bi-phenotypic leukemia; they are more difficult to treat. This is the situation we faced with Tania.

When the results were finalized, I called Miss Brown. Our conversation was uncomfortable; her tone became immediately, though understandably, hostile.

"How'd this happen?" she asked. "Hasn't my daughter been through enough?"

"Tania, Ms. Brown, there is an explanation. The tacrolimus that you take to prevent heart rejection lowers your immune system and makes you more susceptible to developing cancer, frequently lymphoma; leukemia is unusual, but it does sometimes occur."

"No one ever told me that before."

"Well, I'm sorry. Frankly, I'm having difficulty processing the news as well, but one fact is certain—we have to begin anti-leukemia therapy today."

Tania was admitted to Tower 5. Using very simple terms, I explained to her mother what leukemia was in general, and what ambiguous leukemia was specifically. It's not an easy conversation for anyone to comprehend, because it involves speculation and trial and error without the benefit of randomized clinical trials. I explained that initial therapy is directed against acute lymphoblastic leukemia component and we follow the minimal residual disease test (MRD) at the conclusion of the induction phase to determine subsequent treatment. If the MRD is negative and complete remission is attained, treatment continues. If not, we change course. It was not clear to me if Miss Brown or Tania understood anything I said, but they seemed to appreciate the gravity of the situation and signed the consent and assent documents respectively.

Tania spent the next month in the hospital virtually alone; her mother was a no-show. She bonded with her nurses, Melissa White, a child-life specialist, Beth Negles, a social worker, and me for support. She was cheerful, bright, and inquisitive, with soft features and glistening eyes. A prominent scar ran from just above her breastbone to her upper abdomen, a reminder of her previous heart transplant. She was a beautiful young woman, inside and out, and did not deserve such a life of illness and tragedy. She affected me deeply. I was angry, I was sad, I felt helpless, and I was fearful that she would not survive.

I visited Tania often, not only as her officially responsible doctor but also as a friend. If the nurses weren't around, she was usually alone, buried beneath a colorful comforter. She and I began to develop a relationship that transcended the bounds of doctor and patient, and when I would enter her room, she'd sense my presence and sit up in bed, smiling and seeming eager to talk. She told me about high school and her desire to attend Hunter College and study nursing. We talked about how her mother was her best friend, but how Tania was disappointed that she didn't spend nights in the hospital. Tania noticed that virtually every other patient on the floor had a parent or family member staying with them. Why not her mother? She observed that other patients often had family and friends visiting and their rooms were brightly decorated with toys, games, and videos and abundantly replete with food and snacks. Tania's room was stark by comparison, and she was alone.

I rarely allow myself to become personally involved with patients. It's usually not good for me or the patient—there's too much uncertainty. But Tania was different. I was drawn to her—her personality, her smile, her sadness and I suppose I was drawn to the fact that she needed me. Her mother could not be with her, and in some odd way, at that moment in time, I needed to be there for her, not only as a doctor, but as a friend and surrogate parent. Her birth father was not in her life, and her mother never remarried, preferring a revolving door of short-lived relationships with no commitment. This situation left Tania without an older male figure in her orbit—no father, no uncles, no family, no friends.

We talked about everything. We even talked about how, when she would lose her hair, she planned to get a purple wig.

One day Tania asked me, "Dr. Weiner, can I ask you a personal question… something I have been thinking about? I asked Melissa, but she told me I needed to discuss it with you."

I had no idea what Tania could possibly ask me that was so secretive, but knowing she had no one else to turn to, I said, "Of course."

"Are you sure? I haven't even asked my mother. Promise me you won't mention our conversation to anyone."

Hearing this, I was reluctant at first, hesitant to cross the doctor-patient boundary, but I answered, "I'm sure."

Tania told me that she thought she was in love with a senior at Canarsie High School. They had been hanging out together before she became sick, and he wanted to have sex. She told me that she'd had intercourse before, but this was different; she loved him. She realized that things were different now that she had leukemia. She needed my permission.

"What's his name?"

"Tony."

I told Tania she could. In fact, I encouraged her to be with Tony. But I mentioned several caveats that she needed to follow. "Normal blood counts, no signs of infection, and most importantly, he must use a condom. It would be absolutely terrible for your health if you got pregnant. If you follow these simple rules, the answer is yes, just be sensible and careful."

She smiled. "I'll be careful."

After four weeks of initial therapy directed against lymphoblastic leukemia, I performed a bone marrow aspirate including an MRD test to determine remission status. It was positive. I shared the news with Tania and her mother, Tania wearing her purple wig. I told them that the next course of therapy would be directed against the persistent myeloid leukemia cells. The treatment itself consisted of an intense three-drug regimen that would be significantly more aggressive than the previous treatment. The most difficult news was that Tania would be hospitalized for at least an additional three to four weeks, alone. Her sad eyes revealed her disappointment. It was not the treatment or that her leukemia was not in remission that concerned her; it was her strong desire to be with Tony and the forced separation from her boyfriend that caused her extreme consternation. Her emotional pain was palpable.

Tania tolerated the therapy well without any significant adverse reactions and, most importantly, no signs of infection or bleeding. She was in an excellent mood—smiling, talkative, wearing her purple wig; her blood counts were normal and she felt well and strong. We were both optimistic the morning I performed another bone marrow aspirate, four weeks from the start of the second course of chemotherapy. The MRD, disappointingly, remained positive.

Tania was discernably upset but desperately tried to be hopeful. Although I attempted to be stoic, I, too, was visibly upset. Not good. She needed some time at home, to recharge her batteries, physically and psychologically. We discharged her from the hospital and made an appointment to see her in the clinic the following Tuesday. I told her to ask her mother to join and to be prepared to be admitted for another round of chemo.

"Dr. Weiner, can I spend some time with my boyfriend, Tony?"

"Yes, now would be a good time," I told her. "I'll see you next week. Remember the promise you made to be careful and responsible."

She smiled, "No worries, I will. See you Tuesday."

I watched Tania leave the oncology floor. She wore her purple wig, a blue sweatshirt emblazoned with Hunter College across the front, and a pair of jeans with the obligatory holes at the knees. Despite her chagrin with the results of her bone marrow test she seemed content at least for the moment. She would be with Tony.

Tuesday morning came too quickly. Tania and Miss Brown followed me to one of the exam rooms on Irving-7, where mother and daughter sat next to each other, and I positioned myself to face them. I explained that we were not quite where we needed to be. Tania's bone marrow continued to show leukemia blast cells—less than 0.1 percent, but we needed it to be less than 0.01 percent. I suggested we attempt a third round of treatment with very high dose cytarabine and asparaginase, drugs known to be effective against lymphoid and myeloid leukemia. The regimen warranted another long, solitary hospitalization.

"Dr. Weiner, am I gonna be okay?"

"I certainly hope so, Tania, I hope so. Are you ready to get started? I'll walk you over to Tower 5."

Despite being alone again, Tania tolerated the regimen easily with no untoward toxicity. I visited as often as possible. One afternoon as I entered her room, she said, "I have something to tell you, but you can't tell anyone. One afternoon when my mother was at work, Tony came to the apartment. I love him, and I think he loves me too. Promise me I'll get better. I need to be with him."

My heart sank and I was momentarily speechless. I'm not clairvoyant, but I knew the odds of Tania surviving were slim to none. Ambiguous lineage or bi-phenotypic leukemia is difficult to treat—not impossible, but difficult. If patients respond to initial therapy, the odds of survival increase, but Tania did not; her MRD remained positive after two aggressive chemotherapy cycles. Cure would be elusive; not a realistic expectation.

"Promise me," she repeated.

"Tania, we are all doing everything possible."

The day of her next bone marrow test, I sensed that her optimism had been replaced by fear and anxiety; fear and anxiety that the MRD result would be positive; fear and anxiety that the treatments were all to no avail; fear and anxiety that she would not survive.

The bone marrow again betrayed residual leukemic cells, and complete remission remained elusive. We entered uncharted territory.

I explained, "A bone marrow transplant is our ultimate goal. However, to do a transplant without being in remission with a negative MRD is very risky." I told them that I was communicating with leukemia experts from other centers whose opinion I valued to solicit their advice regarding the selection of the next chemotherapy course. I sent an email to Barry Hirsch at the Dana-Farber Cancer Institute in Boston, Karin Kennedy and Will First at New York University, Nerissa Maria Angelo at Memorial Sloan Kettering, Aika Azumi at Lurie Children's in Chicago, and Hon-Ching Shan at St. Jude's in Memphis, Tennessee. The consensus of the surveilled experts was to use a combination of Clofarabine, Etoposide, and Cyclophosphamide. The regimen had been studied by the Children's Oncology Group in a Phase 2 study of children with refractory leukemia, the response rate approached 50 percent, but 25 percent developed veno-occlusive disease, a severe complication of treatment, and died of toxicity.

We discussed Tania during our weekly patient conference on Thursday, but I felt we were throwing shit against the wall to see what would stick. There was no clear regimen that held promise for remission without significant toxicity. We talked about experimental agents, targeted therapies against suspected gene mutations, and the Clofarabine, Etoposide, and Cyclophosphamide idea. Often during such discussions, I thought to myself, *We're talking about Tania. We're talking about a living and breathing child. How can we speak about this so clinically, without emotion? This is life or death.*

Some patients and families, like Tania and her mother, blindly accept whatever their doctor tells them for the sake of time and expediency. However, this blind acceptance places increased pressure on doctors' decision-making and deliberations. I explained to Miss Brown that the regimen had a 50-50 chance of working and that the transplant team, Drs. Krishana and Michels, agreed to initiate the intensive preparatory regimen needed for transplant only if we were able to attain bone marrow aplasia, rather than wait for marrow recovery.

After a few days at home in Brooklyn, Tania was admitted to Tower 5, once again alone, and the five-day regimen began. She tolerated the chemotherapy relatively easily with a low-grade fever, minimal nausea, and stable vital signs, but on day nine, her fourth day of recovery after completing the regimen, the bottom fell out. She became hypotensive with a fever that spiked to 104 and had difficulty breathing.

A RAPID was called to stabilize Tania as quickly as possible at the bedside; she was transported to the 11 Central intensive care unit, where a chest x-ray revealed fluid in her lungs. She had pulmonary edema and ascites, free fluid in her abdomen. She experienced multiple organ failure—heart, lungs, liver, and kidney. Additionally, her bone marrow shut down, and she was extremely pancytopenic with her blood counts in the basement. She developed an overwhelming Aspergillus fungal infection. Survival was doubtful. Medical management had little effect and did not improve her condition. Tania was several weeks shy of her 18th birthday.

I had to have a difficult conversation with Miss Brown. Decisions needed to be made. Standing in Tania's room, we moved to the corner by the window, a view of Broadway below us. I needed to gather myself, exercise restraint, and be professional. I was devastated, but I needed to be grounded and strong. I would grieve in private in my office or at home—not right then.

"Shaneka," I said. "Tania is going to die. There is little hope that she will survive. There's really nothing we can do. Her organs are failing, and she has an untreatable fungal infection. Medical management is not the answer any longer." I paused and asked, "Do you believe in miracles? Are you a religious person?"

"Not really. I do believe in God," she said. "I pray in my own way." She told me that recently she had been asking God to watch over Tania and take care of her. "I guess that's praying."

I told Shaneka that it would take a miracle to save her daughter. I reiterated the fact that medicine was no longer the answer and that there was very little we could do for her. Putting Tania on a respirator would only prolong the inevitable—we needed a miracle.

I told Miss Brown that I had once witnessed a bona fide miracle, and it had made me a believer. "Why not for your daughter?" I asked.

I told her my story from many years ago.

More than 30 years prior, I had taken care of Carlie Logalbo, a teenage girl who had myelogenous leukemia. It was Thanksgiving week, and not unlike Tania, she was deathly ill. She'd had a high fever and was bleeding from every orifice with multiple organ failure. I had been on call that Wednesday evening before the holiday, and I'd had to be the one to tell her mother that her daughter would soon die. I'd said my goodbyes and left the hospital.

Carlie's mother, Melanie, a devout Catholic, spoke with her parish priest, Father Paul, who, in turn, reached out to his old teacher, Cardinal Cooke, who was now the archbishop at St. Patrick's Cathedral in New York City, and told him about Carlie Logalbo. Father Paul arranged a private prayer vigil with the cardinal for that night.

They'd entered the Gothic monolith through the main entrance on Fifth Avenue, and a security guard directed them to the Cardinal's private study behind the main altar of the church.

"Good evening, your Eminence," said Father Paul as he knelt to kiss the cardinal's ring.

"Greetings, my son. This must be Mrs. Logalbo."

"Yes."

"Good evening, your Eminence," said Melanie. "Thank you for seeing us on such short notice, but we don't have much time. The doctors tell me that she is critically ill and could die at any moment. Please help me. Please help Carlie. I beg of you—help us."

"Let us pray together for Carlie," the cardinal replied. "Let us pray for her recovery. Please follow me to my private chapel. Father Paul, please join us. We will pray together. Join me, my child. Tell Christ of Carlie, and ask the Lord to grant her life on this earth."

The devotions lasted not 10 minutes, but Melanie felt renewed strength and courage; it was as if a great weight had been lifted, and although light-headed, she felt free. She thanked Cardinal Cooke, kissed his ring, and bade him goodnight. She and Father Paul traveled home in silence. Melanie returned to the hospital where Carlie was alive but no different. She fell asleep immediately and slept a deep, dreamless night.

Thanksgiving morning, I was in the ICU at 7:30 a.m., alone; the team had not yet formerly gathered for rounds. I noticed several people, nurses, residents, and the critical care fellows outside of Carlie's room, and immediately I rushed to her room, assuming the worst. To my surprise, and to the astonishment of everyone, Carlie was improving—slowly but steadily improving, minute by minute, hour by hour. Her vital signs had stabilized, her medications were withdrawn, her blood count normalized. She was removed from the respirator and the renal dialysis was terminated. What was unfolding before our eyes? Were we witness to a medical miracle?

Friday morning, Carlie was sitting up in bed. "Good morning, Dr. Weiner."

I was speechless. Three days before, I had told the family that I believed Carlie would soon be dead, and there was no path to survival. Today, she was sitting up in bed and saying good morning.

I asked Carlie if she had any memory of what had transpired over the past few days. I asked her if she knew how desperately ill she'd been just a few days before. She told me that she had no memory of the whirlwind of activity that had swept her room over the past few days. She did, however, recall a beautiful dream she'd had. She dreamt that she was surrounded by angels and that Jesus spoke to her.

"Carlie," he had told her. "It is not your time to die and be with me in heaven. You shall live. You shall be well. You shall be a messenger and dedicate your life to helping others less fortunate. You shall be a righteous person."

When we ran the requisite tests, there was no evidence of acute myelogenous leukemia in her blood. I asked Mrs. Logalbo if I could perform a bone marrow test to confirm remission, but she declined. She had all the evidence she needed. We discussed additional therapy, rationalizing that her daughter had not received sufficient treatment to ensure a cure. Again, she declined. Carlie left the hospital about one week after Thanksgiving. She remains well and healthy to this day. She graduated from Notre Dame, became a physical therapist, and married a young man from New Jersey, with whom she's had two children.

Cardinal Cooke passed away several years later. Church scholars had heard of Carlie Logalbo's story and were determined to ascertain whether a miracle had occurred. The Catholic Church launched a movement to beatify Terence Cooke. By canon law, one must perform three documented miracles in order to be designated a saint. I was interviewed by three priests and church scholars, to whom I recounted Carlie's story and near-death experience. I informed them that there was no defined medical explanation for the circumstances surrounding her survival. I told them about Melanie's prayer vigil and audience with the cardinal, and I related Carlie's dream, just as they had told me.

One of the church scholars asked, "Dr. Weiner, in your opinion was this a miracle?"

"Father, your definition of a miracle may differ from mine," I replied. "You and your colleagues must decide if the events rise to that level and withstand liturgical scrutiny. I am a Jewish boy from Brooklyn. All I can tell you is that there is no rational explanation, but only you may determine what is and what is not a miracle."

Shaneka was stunned. "Is it possible? Could Tania survive?"

I had no answer, but instead urged her to stay by Tania's bedside and to pray for her daughter. For the first time in her daughter's care journey, Shaneka stayed over with Tania in her intensive care unit room. She didn't say much but sat with Tania, stroking her hair and gazing at her as only a mother could. When the wrenching decision had to be made, Shaneka agreed that it would be best not to place Tania on a respirator, but rather, to be certain that she was as comfortable as possible. I visited every day and would sit by the side of Tania's bed and speak to her about the goings on around the hospital. She often smiled and grabbed my hand. I whispered, "I am so sorry."

Barely audible, she replied, "Thank you for everything you did for me, thanks for being my friend. But I trusted you. You lied to me. You let me down."

There would be no miracle for Tania. She died peacefully that night with her mother at her side.

I was heartbroken.

Tania affected me as few other patients have moved me. I cared for her deeply, I let her down. Her leukemia was vicious and voracious; it destroyed her. For the moment, it destroyed me too.

＊

BILL OLIVER

Such Promise

We moved the mobile computer to Room 512, Bill Oliver's room. A handwritten sign on the door read, "Sleeping, please respect our quiet time." An understandable request certainly, but one that can never be wholly adhered to in a hospital. I opened the door as quietly and unobtrusively as possible.

"How was Bill's night?" I asked his nurse, Samantha, pleased to see that both Bill and his mother had continued to sleep peacefully.

"He seems comfortable," Samantha replied. "He slept most of the night. The night shift nurses left him alone. They didn't even wake him for vital signs."

"Katie," I said, turning to our pain specialist. "Anything to add?"

"The pain team came by late yesterday afternoon and began tapering the ketamine drip and reducing the dosage of the morphine PCA. They added a fentanyl patch. He's also on methadone orally and oxycodone for breakthrough pain. His pain seems manageable for the moment."

Bill was dying. He was diagnosed with a NUT midline carcinoma, a rare, genetically defined, aggressive, squamous cell epithelial malignancy. It typically affects midline structures, organs in the central core of the body such as sinuses, airways, and chest cavity. It occurs in both children and adults, is resistant to treatment, and is universally fatal with the average survival from diagnosis being less than 12 months. Bill was diagnosed 10 months ago.

Our focus at this time was to find a pain relief regimen that would allow Bill to be discharged in order to receive hospice care at home, where he would be surrounded by his family, his girlfriend, Grace, and his friends from Indian Hills High School. Bill was a very popular student athlete, a member of the soccer team, and one of the best long-distance runners in New Jersey. Everyone in Allendale knew Bill and the Oliver family; everyone knew he had cancer, but few knew the depth and seriousness of his illness.

Getting Bill home would take a village. It would require input from the pain service team, the palliative care team, and the Butterflies Hospice coordinators. The intravenous delivery of narcotics and analgesics used in the hospital is often too complicated for the home setting, so the regimen must be simplified. Finding a routine that Bill's parents, Anne and Steve, could easily manage from home, alongside the visiting nurses from the Butterflies program, would be crucial.

The Olivers were good people. Steve was an attorney in Allendale, New Jersey. He had a small practice which consisted of two partners who managed whatever came through their door, from real estate transactions, to personal injury, to divorce cases. He was a big, affable guy who'd played sports in high school before completing undergraduate and law school at Rutgers, the New Jersey state school. He rarely wore a tie.

Steve was the quiet parent. He listened intently and inscrutably, without apparent judgment. What was most assuredly apparent was his heartbreak at the prospect of losing his son, though he tried his best to remain strong for his wife and, of course, for Bill. In contrast, Anne was visibly emotionally unmoored. She spent every night in the hospital with Bill, accompanied him for every outpatient visit, and was at her son's side when he received his chemotherapy and radiation treatments, when he had difficulty breathing or was unable to sleep because of vomiting, and when he experienced excruciating pain. She was the recipient of all the news—good or bad—first. The burden of Bill's illness fell on her aching shoulders.

Steve arrived at the hospital a few minutes before 10 a.m. There had been an accident on the George Washington Bridge that had the traffic crossing the Hudson River backed up on Route 4 to Queen Anne Road in Teaneck. He arrived almost an hour late and was unnecessarily apologetic.

Bill's primary oncologist, Jacki Blade Gender, was out of town at a meeting, thus, Hanna Carlotay, a pediatric oncology fellow and one of Bill's primary doctors, and I were charged with this important discussion. Hanna is Hungarian, and to this day I have difficulty pronouncing her last name, but that does not diminish the fact that she is an incredible physician. She did her residency at Georgetown University in Washington, D.C., with my friend, Alilah Tarza, who advocated for us to accept her into our fellowship. We did, and Hanna has not been *good*, she has been spectacular. She is the whole package—intelligent, compassionate, soft-spoken yet firm, and the children and families that she cares for adore and trust her; she did not disappoint.

Across from Room 512 there was an alcove with two tables, a banquette, and a water and ice dispenser. It was convenient and close to Bill, should he have awakened from sleep and need his parents.

Anne, Steve, Hanna, and I sat next to each other along the wall. I spread the obligatory papers on the table. "We need to talk about Bill," I began.

"Dr. Weiner—may we call you Michael?"

"Of course, I would prefer if you would."

The Olivers were holding hands. Anne was teary-eyed, a box of Kleenex in her other hand. "Michael, we know Bill is going to die, and in an odd way, he welcomes death. He has suffered more than any teenager should; truly, he has endured almost a year from hell. It will be a blessing for him to be at peace. But he wants to be at home with his family and friends. We need you to promise us that you will make this happen for him."

I promised the Olivers that we would respect their wishes. I assured them that their son would die at home with his family and that we would ensure that he was as comfortable as possible and experienced minimal pain. The pain and palliative care teams would work alongside the Butterflies nurses to find a regimen that would both allow Bill comfort and ensure that he was sufficiently alert to spend as much time as possible with his friends and family. I promised his parents that the social workers, Barbara Klain and Beth Thom, would work with the hospice people to make certain that all of Bill's needs were met.

"We can make this happen quickly," I said. "He will be much more comfortable in a hospital bed, and he'll need a wheelchair, oxygen, and nasogastric-tube feedings for nutrition. Hanna, will you review the medications he will need, including the analgesia cocktail for pain control? Bill is a priority; we will take care of this immediately."

Steve, with his head buried in his hands, looked up and said, "I can't believe this is happening to our son." Holding back the tears, he continued, "He is such a good boy—my best friend really. We don't know how we can live without him."

Hanna moved closer to Anne and Steve and embraced them, "We all love Bill. I am so, so sorry for you," she said.

"We need to have you sign some documents," I said, both hating to force logistics and hoping that practical action might help to ground us all.

The Butterflies hospice program requires that we discuss what we refer to as DNI/DNR (do not intubate/do not resuscitate) ahead of time with the family. What this clarifies is that should Bill's heart stop or his breathing cease, he would not be put on a respirator and he would not receive medication or chest compressions to revive him. Rather, we would let him pass peacefully and without intervention, surrounded by his love ones.

Conversations regarding end-of-life care and DNI/DNR are necessary, if painful, discussions. They are never easy, and in the case of a child or young adult, they are excruciating, but they are vitally important for all concerned in order to assure that, in the event of a significant decline, the desires of the patient and family are respected and adhered to without question. It is an imperative directive for the residents and nurses caring for the patient.

For a medical professional, it is also a mandatory document to have in your possession when a patient passes. The local police department and the funeral home will need documentation that Bill was cared for at Columbia, that he had cancer, that he was receiving hospice care, and that his death was expected.

"I am so sorry to have to have this conversation with you," I said, fighting back tears. "Please forgive me, but preparation now will make a huge difference in the future."

The four of us were sobbing. I wiped away the moisture from my eyes with the sleeve of my shirt. I repositioned the documents that needed to be signed on the table and took a pen from my shirt pocket and handed it to Steve.

Without uttering a word or making a comment, he scanned the papers in front of him. "Tell me where to sign."

He printed BILL EDWARD OLIVER at the top of the page on the blank line indicating the name of the patient. Where the document asked, "Has your physician explained the meaning of Do Not Intubate and Do Not Resuscitate and have your questions been answered?" Steve indicated yes and first printed and then signed his name, STEVEN OLIVER. Hanna signed as the witness, and I signed as the responsible doctor. I handed the completed document to Carolyn Manacia, the senior nurse administrator, to be included in the permanent patient record.

Legally, Bill was not a minor, having recently celebrated his 18th birthday, and Steve, Anne, Hanna, and I all recognized that he must be involved in what had just transpired.

We entered Room 512 together. Bill was awake.

"Good morning, Bill," I said.

"Hey, Dr. Weiner."

I moved close to the hospital bed and extended my hand. Bill grasped my right hand with all the strength he could muster. It was his routine to shake hands with a firm grip, an indication that he was well. No matter how ill he felt, his handshake was strong. Bill appeared pale and gaunt; his 6-foot, 2-inch frame was horribly cachectic with no muscle mass. End-stage unremitting cancer steals the body of shape and form; there is a distinct similarity among cancer patients at the end of life—skin, bones, sunken eyes, pallor, and tremulous voices. Death was not far away, but near.

Bill was dying.

"Are you comfortable this morning?" Hanna asked. "How is your pain?"

Anne sat on the bed, and moved closer to her son, caressing his beautiful bald head. Steve stood at the foot of the bed, and I pulled a chair close to Bill and his mother.

Bill told us that his pain was a 5 out of 10—tolerable. He told us that the minor changes made to the new pain regimen that Dr. Gordon and the pain team had devised were helping. He told us that he was comfortable and more alert.

I explained to Bill that Hanna and I had just had a discussion with his parents, and we wanted to tell him what we were talking about. I told Bill, "We want to send you home to be with your family and friends. Our main concern is that we want you to be as pain free as possible, and I think we are almost there—it appears that the minor changes to the regimen are working effectively. You know that Jacki Blade Gender is away, but we communicated with her and she agrees with this plan. Hanna, the nurses, and social workers are making the final arrangements, and the Butterflies team are prepared for you at home."

I told Bill and his parents that, before she went out of town, Dr. Blade Gender suggested that we begin a new chemotherapy drug called Vorinostat. It is taken orally every day for 14 days, and we can then determine whether to continue or not. It has very few side effects, and Bill should tolerate it without any difficulty. JBG is an expert in novel drugs, and she thought it might help.

Jacki had also recognized that offering a terminally ill patient chemotherapy sends a message of hope and allows them to believe that their doctor has not given up. If there is 1 chance in 100 or 1 in 1,000, why not Bill?

"What do you think, do you want to give it a try?"

Bill hardly looked up. "I really don't see the point. It has no chance of working, and I'm just fed up. I'm sick of trying things that are really just a charade to make my parents feel better." He sighed. "Will it make me nauseated? Does it have any side effects?"

"Probably not," I replied. "How about giving it a try and if it makes you uncomfortable or causes any other untoward effects, I promise we can stop it. Give it a chance."

Without looking up, Bill took a slow, deep breath. He was too tired to fight with me. "Okay," he said with resignation. "As long as I can stop it when I want to."

I told Bill and his parents that we were quite certain that all the details for discharge could be completed by the next day and we could have him home by the weekend.

"I think your father is going home soon to meet the delivery driver," I said. "Everything you need, a hospital bed, oxygen, all your meds, IV poles, and feeding tubes will be waiting for you when you arrive tomorrow. Your father said that he is setting up the family room on the first floor with all your supplies. That way you can be near your family. Hanna and Dr. Blade Gender will see you in clinic on Tuesday, a routine visit, to be certain that all is well."

"Thanks," Bill murmured, his eyes beginning to close. "I'm going to rest a bit, the medicine's making me tired, and I think my friends are visiting this afternoon."

Bill was always polite and gracious; that was just who he was. But today, he was unusually calm and resigned. He had endured hell on earth since his diagnosis. Was he angry? Certainly. Was he sad? To be sure. But he was fatalistic and accepting of his plight; relieved to be going home.

Anne was numb, on another planet, but knowing that Bill would soon be home helped to lighten that burden.

Steve gave his son a hug, kissed his forehead, and told him he would be back that afternoon with his sister Elizabeth.

Turning to Anne, he said a quick goodbye. "Do you need anything from home? I'll call you in a few hours."

Heavily medicated, Bill quickly fell asleep. With Steve gone home to set things up with the Butterflies Hospice crew at their home in Allendale, Anne stared at her son as only a mother could.

I moved to the window and looked at the rooftops across 165th Street and Broadway. After a time, Anne joined me. As I gazed into her eyes, I observed an all too familiar sight: a parent experiencing unimaginable, indescribable sadness and defeat. Despite her prayers and presumably the best that modern medicine had to offer, she had failed, we had failed to save her son.

Every child's life is special and its loss tragic, but Bill had developed a special place in my heart. I, too, felt extraordinary despair. Everyone who knew him felt loss; it was palpable.

Cutting through my thoughts, Anne asked me, "Can we talk for a few minutes?"

"Sure," I replied. "We've finished rounds, let me tell the team where I am in case they need me."

Anne paused. I worried that I had pushed her. Perhaps, as the mother of a dying child, Anne was hoping to distract herself. But when she looked up at me, her eyes shining, I saw relief. "My goodness," she said. "There is so much to tell. I remember when Bill was diagnosed as if it were yesterday. Are you certain you have time?"

"Yes, of course."

Anne told me that in the fall of 2016, the Indian Hills High School boys soccer team had a season like no other, with a final record of 22-0, winning the county, sectional, and state championships—the coveted "triple crown." Bill was a junior and started as midfielder, contributing five goals and six assists over the course of the season. The rigorous high school soccer season blended into winter and then spring track, with no breaks. Distance running, the mile and two-mile, were his best events, and he excelled. Bill was running eight miles every day and competing in meets multiple times a week. He was excited to reach his new goal, a 4-minute, 15-second mile. College track coaches had been reaching out to Bill for a few months, and they were all excited by his potential. His dream was to run the mile for the University of Pennsylvania.

He was training with grit and determination, but in March, he started to feel like his body was not responding the way it should. Throughout the winter, indoor track season, and the beginning of spring track, Bill had stopped achieving the times he had been striving for and had begun to grow frustrated with his performance. He told his coaches that his legs felt heavy. Keenly aware of his body, he'd said that he didn't feel like he was taking in oxygen like he used to. He was treated for allergies but found no relief. His allergist gave him an inhaler to treat what his doctors thought might be exercise-induced asthma. His sister had asthma, so it seemed reasonable.

At a county meet in mid-May, Bill stepped off of the track during the two-mile race. He was complaining of severe chest pain and difficulty breathing and had a blinding pain in his right cheek and eye.

Anne related that she and Steve took Bill to the Emergency Room at Valley Hospital for an x-ray where they were told that there was a cloud in Bill's right lung. He was diagnosed with pneumonia. However, two weeks later, he was not responding to antibiotics, and his symptoms were worsening. We brought Bill back to the hospital emergency room.

She remembered thinking in retrospect that this day changed their lives forever. Anne said, "The doctors repeated the chest x-ray and determined that the cloud in Bill's lung was larger than a few weeks earlier and suggested an immediate CT scan."

"Steve, Bill, and I waited," she said. "The minutes turned to hours; the hours felt like days."

She paused, contemplating, before continuing, "We had no idea that a bomb was about to explode; a bomb that would detonate in our son's chest cavity; a bomb that would leave a crater and throw our family into the bottom of the abyss."

Anne recalled that the Emergency Room doctor came to Bill's room and asked to speak with Steve and me outside in the hall. We left Bill alone for a moment and met the doctor in the hallway, just outside his room. The doctor told us that the CT scan showed three malformed tumors in Bill's chest: one in his right lung and two more in his chest cavity. He told us that the malformed nature of the tumors was an indicator of cancer and that the radiologist thought the most likely preliminary diagnosis was lymphoma.

"'I'm so sorry,' he had said."

Anne told me that she had become overcome with horror and felt detached from reality. She had difficulty seeing clearly and couldn't breathe. She remembered she grabbed onto Steve with all her strength. It was all she could do to hold herself up. She told me Steve was a rock, remained completely calm, and asked pointed questions with incredible clarity. The next thing she knew, her legs buckled, everything went black. She remembered needing something to hold onto, so she labored toward an empty gurney nearby to stabilize herself. Anne continued to tell me that a nurse took her arm, guided her into a chair in an empty lounge, knelt at her feet, grabbed her by the sides of her shoulders, and spoke clearly, yet compassionately.

"'I am so sorry this is happening, but you *have* to focus on your son.'"

I was amazed. "Anne, your memory for detail is incredible. Did you keep a diary, write things down? My goodness."

She shook her head. "Michael, Bill is my life, my first born. Our bond is special, our relationship unique. I am able to summon every detail, every incident, every conversation. There is so much more. I could talk forever about Bill. Are you doing okay on time?" she asked, looking at my watch automatically.

Reluctant to deprive Anne of this moment, one that was so important to her, I said, "Yes, of course. If they need me, they know where to find me."

Gazing at her son asleep in bed, Anne said, "Thank you. This is important to me, to be able to talk about Bill."

She continued where she left off, telling me that she and Steve had discussed and weighed their options. A decision had to be made quickly and thoughtfully.

Anne recalled feeling sick, how she had almost fainted, was furious with herself, embarrassed. She told me that two nurses rolled a gurney to the doorway of the lounge and helped her onto it. After a few minutes of lying down, she was able to catch her breath and regain her composure. As she walked into Bill's room and saw her son's expression, she began to laugh. She didn't want him to see her upset. This wasn't the first time she'd fainted in a medical environment; it had become something of a family joke, she was certain it wouldn't be the last.

"I remember saying to Bill, 'Sorry, honey, I was just looking for a little attention, you know me.'"

She reminisced how she and Steve had smiled at Bill, their sweet little boy, and before she knew it, words were coming out of her mouth. "You're not going to believe this," she said. "But it looks like you may have tumors in your chest. They think it may be cancer."

She continued, "The words were out before I had time to think about them or give them shape. My tone remained inappropriately light-hearted—almost manic. 'How crazy is that?' I said, beginning to laugh mechanically.

"Steve, ever calm, took charge, telling Bill that we would have to go to another hospital for tests and care, we would be heading to Columbia that night. Incredibly, Bill took everything in stride and was calm, cool, and collected—the way he has always processed everything.

"Finding out that Bill had cancer brought us to a dark, desperate, and exceedingly painful place. Distraught and paralyzed with shock and fear, we were forced into a world that we wish didn't exist for any parent; a world where we were forced to face our own child's mortality.

"Bill was taken by ambulance to the emergency room at the Morgan Stanley Children's Hospital at Columbia University Medical Center. We knew that it was one of the best places for Bill and felt secure at least that he would get the care he needed."

Anne told me she rode in the ambulance with Bill, and Steve managed to harness the strength and sanity to follow in his car. "To this day, I have no idea how Steve made that drive."

Bill was uncomfortable in the ambulance. The tumors in his chest were causing so much discomfort and pressure on his airway that he could not lie flat without pain. He had difficulty breathing and complained of a blinding pain on the right side of his face.

We arrived at Columbia at 10:30 at night. The hallway ramp made it difficult to keep Bill's gurney from rolling too far ahead. He was triaged at a portable computer station, and rolled down the ramp and into room number 23, where he began to vomit uncontrollably from the morphine he had been given to manage his pain during the ambulance trip. He couldn't lie flat without severe pain and respiratory distress. The head of his bed was elevated to make it easier for him to breathe, and he was given oxygen and pain and nausea medication through an IV catheter inserted into his right forearm.

Anne recalled thinking that the emergency room seemed like Grand Central Station. It was packed with crying children, parents trying to comfort them, and doctors and nurses trying to keep calm and do the best they could to attend to the needs of the overflowing masses.

She went on to say that the first person they met at Columbia was a tall, slender doctor in his early 30s.

"'Hi, I'm Dr. Kenny. You must be Bill. You look like a runner. Are you a runner, Bill?' he asked. Bill nodded. 'You look just like me long and lean.'

"I remember that Steve and I were relieved by Dr. Kenny's tranquil demeanor in the face of such devastating news. My antennae were up and my senses heightened during this period of intense emotion. Things were unfolding at a rapid pace, and I remember feeling like I was trapped in a vortex, spiraling out of control.

"Dr. Kenny examined and assessed Bill, talking to him as if they'd met in a park on a beautiful day. He told us that it would be best to admit Bill to the pediatric intensive care unit where he would be safer, as patients in the PICU receive concentrated, one-on-one nursing care.

"The attendants pushed Bill's bed onto the elevator at the front entrance of the emergency room on the ground floor of the building. There was room in the elevator for Steve and me as well, so we climbed aboard. As the doors opened onto the ninth floor, I was stunned. It was the middle of the night—3:30 a.m.—but the activity in the unit was frenetic; despite the hour, it seemed like the middle of the day. The floor was filled with people in uniform—doctors, young and old, nurses in scrubs, and respiratory therapy technicians, and there were lights flashing and *beep, beep, beep* sounds coming from every room. I could hardly begin to take it all in.

"Bill's room was in the corner, number 901. My first impression was that the room looked more like a fishbowl than a room. A wall of glass stood between Bill's bed in the center of the space and the nurses' station. A desk, chair, and computer were pressed up against the glass facing into the room, where Bill's nurses would sit to monitor him day and night.

"The windows on the back wall, which did not open, looked out to the buildings across Broadway. Bill's bed was surrounded by machines and IV poles. Next to the bed was a faux leather armchair that could unfold into a small bed, and which Steve and I would take turns sleeping in for the next few weeks; but that first night in the PICU, we did not sleep."

Anne paused and looked up at me. "It's incredible how vivid my memories of those first hours and days still are," she said. "It's like it happened yesterday," she said, her face crumpling. "Every day I wake up and pray that it never happened at all; that this is just some awful nightmare."

Standing next to Anne, I knew there was very little I could say. Medicine had failed, our work as doctors, had little chance of success from day one. Strangely, I think Steve, Anne, and Bill knew that all along.

Her son would die, and there was nothing that either of us could do about it. I put my hand on Anne's shoulder, and for a moment we stood together in silence, gazing out the window, reflecting on the remarkable life of Bill Oliver.

Maybe, Just Maybe

M y cell phone beeped with a message from Danica. "Ariella Colon is ready to be discharged and Mrs. Colon has a few questions. Can you speak to her for a few minutes?"

"Of course, I'll be right there. Anne please excuse me, I need a few minutes."

Bill woke from his narcotic induced sleep, "Mom, can you rub my back?"

Arrangements had been made with Bill's pain management team and the Butterflies hospice nurses, Bill was ready to be home. The Butterflies team was set, and welcomed him home to Allendale. His weekend was better than anyone could have hoped for. He was mostly pain free, and was even able to eat a pepperoni pizza, at least a slice. He took the Vorinostat every day without any untoward effects, and was inundated with visitors, family and friends. Bill's spirits were high.

Ten days later, a Tuesday morning, at 9 a.m. the elevator door on Irving Pavilion seventh floor opened, Bill had arrived by ambulance for a scheduled check-up, his mom at his side. It was mid-December, the weather in New York was cold and gray, Bill was wrapped in blankets, the EMT techs wheeled his stretcher to the reception area. Bill insisted on standing and walking by himself to one of the large, blue, reclining lounge chairs in the cage. He moved slowly, tentatively, but by himself. He settled in for the day. Carol Terri, one of the outpatient nurses greeted Bill, placed his hospital ID band on his right wrist, took his vital signs: blood pressure, pulse rate, temperature. She passed on height and weight. The Butterflies nurse left his PORT accessible, but capped. Carol cleaned the hub with betadine solution, attached a syringe to draw his blood work: a complete blood count, chemistries, and a type and cross should he need a blood transfusion. Dr. Blade Gender would see him, complete an exam, check his results, and deal with any issues.

I walked to his lounge chair, "Hey, Bill. How are you today?"

He extended his right hand and gripped mine to give me that firm Bill Oliver hand shake and said, "Can't complain."

"Good morning, Anne. How was the weekend?"

"The weekend was fantastic, Bill was comfortable, had a house full of friends, practically the entire Indian Hills High School soccer team stopped by. His girlfriend Grace joined us for dinner on Saturday night and then Sunday, Steve and Bill watched the Giants game. It was joyful to all be together."

"That's great to hear," I said, and I meant it. The entire hospital staff was fond of Bill, and though I wasn't his primary attending, I'd grown particularly attached after Anne had opened up to me and recounted the first few days of his diagnosis. My heart ached for the Olivers and though I knew there was little we could do to help, I was committed to doing whatever was possible, even if all that was possible was lending an ear and hearing Anne's memories. "I have a few meetings, I'll be back around 11. Let's try to catch up."

"I'd like that, we'll speak later. I want to get Bill settled for the day. He has something to tell you as well."

When the outpatient clinic was originally renovated, virtually all patient treatments were administered in the infusion area in the southwest corner of the seventh floor an area with floor to ceiling windows; however, as the volume of new patients grew significantly we needed to increase the number of treatment stations. Thus, the cage. When the clinic was first constructed the space was an adolescent library and secondary waiting area, now it resembled the ring in a kickboxing arena with metal poles and netting. It's an eyesore, but functional; it provides an additional 12 treatment locations all with reclining dark blue loungers.

Bill's labs resulted before 10 a.m. He was anemic, his platelet count was dangerously low, and his serum sodium was well outside the normal range, not unexpected. Bill needed help: transfusions of red blood cells and platelets as well as hydration with normal saline. He would be in clinic all day.

When I returned to the seventh floor at 11:15 Bill was resting comfortably, dozing in and out of sleep Carol administered morphine to blunt his pain and Benadryl and Tylenol as premeds before the blood transfusions to prevent a transfusion reaction.

Turning to Anne I asked, "Are you up to chatting for a bit?"

"Sure, I'd like that if you have the time."

Anne stood and walked to a chair close to the computer desk on the far wall of the cage. She was teary-eyed thinking about that day, the worst day of her life, the day that had changed Bill's life, and the lives of the entire Oliver family, forever. Gone was any gleeful anticipation about her son's future, high school graduation, proms, college, sports, girls, marriage, and law school to cancer, and certain death.

I asked Anne if she wanted privacy, but she wanted to be close to Bill if he needed her. I moved a chair to the computer desk and sat across from her. She began speaking in a soft, quivering voice. Her memory for detail was extraordinary.

She told me her fear was far greater than her curiosity and knew she couldn't manage any more fear so decided not to Google "NUT midline carcinoma." She articulated how she needed to regain her strength and harness hope to help Bill get through this. She became laser focused on coaching Bill through anything and everything that was to come. Steve, on the other hand was determined to learn as much as he could about this horrific disease. He spent hours on the computer reading everything available. He called my brother John, a gastroenterologist at the Cleveland Clinic. They spoke daily, often many times a day, Steve asking questions, seeking opinions and advice. He also reached out to Dr. Cristof Berlin, a pathologist at Harvard who is studying this cancer. Steve was arming himself with knowledge in order to forge ahead.

I listened intently.

Anne conveyed to me a dilemma that she and Steve faced, "We knew we had to have a conversation with Bill, but were at a loss determining what to tell him."

"He is an intelligent, resourceful 17-year-old. Surely, he needed to know why he was so sick, why he had two surgical biopsies of his lungs, why he was in pain and why he was having difficulty breathing. This would not be easy. Do we tell him the truth or talk around reality? How do we tell him he has a rare and frankly incurable cancer? Steve and I realized the conversation would be near impossible."

She recalled going into his room to speak to Bill, sitting on the bed next to him while Steve stood in the background. Jacki Blade Gender told him that he had a very unusual type of cancer called a NUT midline carcinoma. His immediate reaction was to ask, "What kind of NUT? Walnuts, almonds, pecans?"

Anne mentioned that Bill's humor broke the ice and made the rest of the conversation easier and that Jacki told us she had a plan for treatment that involved aggressive chemotherapy followed by surgery and perhaps radiation therapy as well. She told Bill that as the treatment began to work and kill the tumor cells, he would feel better, the pain would lessen significantly, his breathing would return to normal, and his strength would improve. She asked Bill if he had any questions, he did not. He seemed to believe that if he did what the doctors asked him to do and followed instructions, he would be fine and cured. "We signed a consent form for chemotherapy and Bill signed an assent document. Treatment began that very night."

"I also refused to do any reading or research, I believed through sheer necessity and force of will that if we followed the doctors' instructions that we would beat this thing. Steve of course knew better, he knew that Bill's chances of survival were next to none, that treatment might slow things down or improve Bill's quality of life, but that ultimately it was hopeless. Still, we had to try.

"Dr. Blade Gender set Bill on a course of the most aggressive treatment possible. The regimen had been reported by the Scandinavians to have activity in NUT midline carcinomas, although the number of patients in the report was small. The regimen resembled the treatment used for Ewing's sarcoma; it included six different chemotherapy drugs to be given for the first five days of each cycle, with the cycles lasting 21 days. Days 6 through 21 were for recovery, Jacki planned to administer 12 cycles. Jacki provided us with information about the side effects of the chemotherapy drugs. We asked Bill if he wanted to read the material but he declined. I initially declined as well; I knew friends from the neighborhood who had gone through chemotherapy, the drugs ravaged their bodies and brought them to their knees. Was this what my son would face. I recall being terrified, but I wanted no details. What would it change, absolutely nothing? What was the point? Steve on the other hand read every word on every page about every drug. He was scared senseless. The drugs had both short- and long-term toxicities: damage to the kidneys and heart, allergic reactions, liver problems, and on and on. What comfort he derived from this information was a mystery to me, but that's Steve.

"Bill's doctors and nurses kept a close eye on him throughout chemo infusions, checking his vitals every half hour for the duration of the administrations. On the third night of chemo he developed a fever, his blood pressure dropped dangerously low. A RAPID CODE, an indication that a patient's vital signs are abnormal, was called, he was rushed to the ICU, started on antibiotics and hyperhydration with fluids. He responded and improved quickly, within a day and a half, he stabilized and returned to the pediatric oncology floor to complete round one. The chemo made Bill sick to his stomach, temporarily sapped his strength, and caused a great deal of pain in his chest. Jacki told us that it was possible the chest pain was an indication that the drugs were working and the cancer cells were being destroyed. We had hope."

Anne told me that she never allowed Bill to be alone. How she was deathly afraid that he would Google the name of his tumor, learn about its rarity, and read that it is tantamount to a death sentence; she contemplated how he could possibly process that he was going to die. She conveyed to me how she was determined to remain positive, to maintain a hopeful attitude, and attempt to return to a normal life, but of course that this was virtually impossible. The reality was that Bill had an untreatable cancer. He was going to die. That's all there is to it, he was going to die.

Anne paused for a moment to take a deep breath. Those words, "He is going to die," would never get easier. She gazed straight ahead and I wondered if she was even aware of my presence. It was clear that she needed to talk, to relive those first days and memories, to go over what had happened in an attempt to make sense of it, though of course it would never make sense, childhood cancer is fundamentally senseless.

She began to speak again.

"The days following chemotherapy were different, difficult, but different. Prior to treatment Bill had been in pain and had difficulty breathing. Post therapy he was weak, had unrelenting nausea, and vomiting. He'd lost significant weight, and just wanted so badly to go home."

"Soon, Bill, soon," Jacki told him. "You're almost there."

Anne remembered feeling joyful when slowly, ever so slowly Bill improved, his appetite increased, he was able to eat a bowl of pasta, chicken, a baked potato. She told me how he walked around the fifth floor pushing his IV pole for exercise. A red cell transfusion improved his stamina and the pain was less.

"Finally, three and a half weeks after being admitted he was discharged. We left the oncology floor with Bill in a wheelchair and as I wheeled him past the nurse's station into the elevator lobby we could hear cheering and clapping. The doctors and nurses gathered in the lobby with noise makers, horns and silly string to celebrate Bill's discharge; he chuckled and with a huge smile on his face and waved goodbye."

Anne paused for a moment, "I want you to know how grateful I am to you for being such a good listener, it is therapeutic for me to recount and tell Bill's journey."

"Bill's first days back at home were wonderful, I had an entirely new perspective and the only thing that mattered was being home with Bill and having our family together under one roof. It was simply the greatest thing in the world. From morning to night our house was filled with Bill's friends, the soccer team, Bill Breck, the track coach, and several of his teachers. We felt a whole new sense of peace and completeness that we had never felt before. Bill was calm and never once mentioned his cancer. He talked about school, running the mile, girls, and pizza. His coping mechanism was to live outside of reality, to deny he was sick, to talk about what all his friends talked about and never, not once mention NUT midline carcinoma. He had a healthy appetite, good energy, and was sleeping well. His pain was gone and his breathing was strong. The chemotherapy was doing something. He soon lost his hair and shaved his head completely bald.

"Dr. Blade Gender was happily surprised by Bill's quick recovery from the effects of chemotherapy and decided that Bill could handle 'kicking his treatment up a notch.' In an aggressive move, she changed his chemotherapy from three-week cycles to two-week cycles. This meant that Bill would lose a week of recovery time . . . cutting his time at home from 16 days down to 9 days.

"It's going to be brutal, but we need to be aggressive if we want to have any chance of beating this thing," Dr. Blade Gender said. "The chemotherapy will knock the crap out of him and as soon as he is feeling better we'll do it again."

"I recall thinking, *Holy shit, will this really be my son's life?*

"Bill did not want to talk about his illness or his treatments, at least not with us. He told us that he did not Google NUT midline carcinoma, and while we didn't believe him, we also chose not to press him.

"He told us what we wanted to hear, he said, 'I trust Dr. Blade Gender and as long as I do what they tell me to do they said I would be okay, what else is there to say? What choice do I have?'"

I listened as Anne told me that she did everything in her power to protect Bill. She indicated that she filtered, or at least tried to screen conversations, how she was desperate to shield him from anything that would diminish his hope and spirit. In so doing so, she forced him to exist in a fantasy world. Everyone knew that Bill would not be alright; he had a malicious, unrelenting cancer, one that would prevent him from living his dreams. He would not attend the senior prom with Grace, he would not graduate from high school, win the state mile championship, run in the Penn Relays, attend the University of Pennsylvania, or become a lawyer like his father. In a sense Bill had been deprived of coming to grips with his reality and honestly sharing his deepest, innermost thoughts and fears.

"Chemotherapy is the ultimate double-edged sword. It was apparently having some positive effect, Bill's pain was practically gone, his voice stronger and between treatments he was able to be with friends and even go to the Jersey Shore, he always loved the beach at Point Pleasant and body surfing in the Atlantic Ocean. But just as they seemed to help, the treatment knocked the living shit out of him. During the five days of chemotherapy and the two to three days thereafter, Bill experienced horrible nausea and vomiting, body and bone pain, and extreme weakness. If nothing else, Bill was resilient. Between chemotherapy admissions he would try to build himself up, sleep and recuperate at home before repeating the process over again. We had a routine treatment, nine days at home with clinic visits on Tuesdays and Fridays."

Out of her right eye, Anne noticed Bill stirring.

"I'm right here, honey. What do you need? Do you want something to eat or drink?"

"No, not now. I think I want to get on my laptop and answer some emails and maybe watch the episodes of *Game of Thrones* that I missed."

We moved a portable table close to Bill, propped him up in his reclining chair, and I plugged his laptop into a wall outlet behind him.

"Thanks."

"To be continued," Anne said to me, "I need to be with Bill."

"Of course."

The rest of the day proved uneventful. Kim Bono, an outpatient nurse practitioner on the solid tumor group spoke with the Butterflies hospice team to be certain that everything was addressed for Bill's return home. The EMT ambulance team arrived at 4:30, Bill insisted on a wheelchair.

"No stretcher, guys."

He sat in the wheelchair and his nurses wrapped him in blankets and pushed him to the elevators. "See you Friday," he said as the doors opened and he and his mom disappeared from view.

Friday was similar to Tuesday. Bill arrived on a stretcher and walked to the same dark blue recliner, had his vital signs taken, and labs drawn. As expected he needed blood and platelets, and the premeds added to his existing narcotic regimen put him to sleep. Carol sent me a message telling me Bill was here and Mrs. Oliver was looking for me. I messaged back, "Be right there."

"Good morning, how are things?"

"Stable, he's comfortable. The Butterflies nurses are great."

Anne and I retreated to the computer desk as Bill dozed.

She handed me a copy of an email that she had sent to friends and family.

> *Thank you ALL so much for your notes, cards, gifts, your visits and your kindness. Thank you for making us dinner, buying us food, cutting our grass and washing our clothes. Thank you for sending us gift cards, cleaning our home, stocking and cleaning our fridge and checking in on Paul and Elizabeth. Thank you for your referrals, connections and offers of assistance. Thank you for your phone calls, texts, notes and emails. Most of all, thank you ALL for your constant thoughts and prayers. We are so blessed by the overwhelming and unending love and support from family, friends and our community. This is what gives us the strength to wake up every day and fight with hope and faith in our hearts. Love and support + faith and hope + brilliant and compassionate medical care = a CURE. We are humbled and grateful beyond words.*

The ravages of having a child with cancer do not begin and end with that child. The disease not only effects the patient, parents, siblings, family, and friends, but also an entire community. It takes a village.

"I've been overwhelmed by the outpouring of kindness," Anne told me. "As devastating as this experience has been, the small silver lining has been seeing how truly supported we are. I had no idea how many friends we truly had."

I told Anne I was pleased to hear this. "I am not, however, surprised," I told her. "I know how devasting having a child with cancer can be and the outpouring of your community does not surprise me. Are you up to talking today?"

"Yes, I have actually been looking forward to it. You know, talking about Bill and recounting his story helps tremendously. I appreciate you listening."

Anne kept an extensive diary and was able to pick up where she left off the last time we spoke. She told me that in mid-July, Bill completed two cycles of poisons, but actually felt good, considering all he had experienced. "He had his first CT scan since therapy began to assess its effects. The results of the scan would tell us how the tumors were responding to treatment and would assist Bill's doctors and surgeons in determining a surgical course of action. With our fingers crossed and our breath held, the final reading found that all three tumors had shrunk over 50 percent."

She recalled that Jacki told us this was reason to celebrate. "It was a huge milestone, a positive response after only two rounds of chemotherapy indicated that Bill was responding well, that his body was fighting and the treatments were working. Bill had been as strong, positive and hopeful as any human being could possibly be."

"Bill was, of course, beyond ecstatic with the news, which doubtless made round three of chemotherapy his most tolerable to date. He had no symptoms, none. He was in great spirits, watching movies, laughing and eating everything in sight. It was a beautiful summer day and we spent an hour and a half walking through the hospital gardens, his IV pole in tow. We sat together on a bench in the shade and enjoyed the sunshine, the breeze and each other. The day was a gift." Anne glowed. She was in awe of Bill; he was truly her hero.

"Jacki Blade Gender told us that if Bill's response to round three of chemotherapy was good, surgery would be the next step followed by radiation therapy. His response was not good, it was great. We were excited to meet Jordan Klein, Chief of Thoracic Surgery, but we were shocked by how young he looked. We soon learned looks are deceiving, he was older and significantly more experienced than his appearance told. In fact, reading his resume on Google revealed a surgeon of extraordinary skill.

"Dr. Klein was terrific, he was reassuring to Bill and he lived in Ridgewood, New Jersey, the neighboring town to our home in Allendale. We liked him immediately. Surgery would be scheduled for late August. We felt both exhilarated and scared out of our minds. Surgery is definitive, if the cancer could be removed, maybe just maybe, Bill would be able to beat the odds and survive. Maybe, just maybe, Bill would once again play soccer, break records running the mile and two-mile races. Maybe, just maybe, our prayers would be answered.

"Bill was energized. He did a remarkable job navigating this unimaginable experience while trying to maintain a positive attitude and an energetic spirit. He told Steve that he was excited about the surgery, that he would do anything and gladly give up his body for a chance to be cured. His sense of humor was a source of strength; and he had a knack for making others relax. Throughout his ordeal, he often reminded us that, 'Everything happens for a reason.'

"The morning of surgery, August 28th, Bill, Steve and I were up at 4:30 in the morning. We showered quickly, skipped breakfast and drove to New York Presbyterian for a 5:30 check in. At that hour, traffic on the George Washington Bridge was light and we arrived early. We entered the hospital through the Milstein Hospital Building on Fort Washington Avenue, valet parked the car and proceeded to the third floor Milstein Heart Hospital for registration.

"'You must be Bill Oliver,' said Maria Vasquez, the registrant smiling pleasantly.

"'Yes, I am.'

"'We've been expecting you. Dr. Klein's office called and told us you were a special young man and I can see that they were right. They told us to extra special care of you. We know this is a big day and we are all praying for you. Dr. Klein is incredible, you are in excellent hands.' Maria handed us a clipboard with several documents including consents, health care proxies, insurance confirmation forms. Steve scanned them. He didn't have the head to read them carefully; it was too late for that. He signed them all."

The Milstein Heart Hospital was the newest building on the medical center campus, it's a glass and steel, circular building that connects the Irving Pavilion to the older Milstein Hospital Building, the main inpatient building for the Columbia University Medical Center and New York Presbyterian Hospital. The Heart Hospital is a multi-purpose clinical facility that also serves as the pre-operative check-in area for the operating rooms in the main hospital.

Anne recalled that they directed them to proceed to station five where they greeted by Kathy Schaeffer, "'Good morning Bill, we've been expecting you, how are you feeling this morning?' she asked.

"'Ok, I guess.'

"No jokes today from Bill, he was anxious about surgery. How could he not be nervous? His chest was about to be cracked open, his life was on the line. Holy crap, I was petrified as well. I took some deep breaths and prayed that I would not faint. I forced myself to hold it together.

"Kathy handed Bill two hospital gowns and instructed him to put the first one on, opened to the back, and the second one over the first, opened to front. Bill changed and placed his clothes in a large white plastic bag with a draw string marked 'Personal Belongings, New York Presbyterian Hospital.' He handed Steve his wallet, watch, and keys. He jumped onto the stretcher and Kathy took his vital signs, and asked the obligatory questions about allergies and medications, etc.

"Dr. Klein arrived at 7 a.m., 'Good morning, Bill.'

"He told us that he planned to make a large incision along Bill's right rib cage in order to remove the lower lobe of Bill's right lung to fully extract the tumor. The remainder of the surgery was dependent upon a number of factors, but it was his plan to remove the other two tumors completely, as well as all of the lymph nodes in Bill's thorax. It would require work, but Dr. Klein's aim was to leave Bill cancer free, if at all possible. The entire operation was estimated to take about five hours, give or take. Steve signed the consent for surgery—I was terrified, shaking like a leaf. Unfortunately, it is my nature to always see the worst, the dark side. I wish it weren't so, but it is my nature and there was certainly nothing I could do about it that morning. I prayed harder than I have ever prayed before, 'Please dear God protect my son even if the surgery is not successful, please allow him to survive the operation.'"

Anne paused, regaining her breath. Until now, I had listened closely but done very little to participate in conversation. It seemed vital to Anne that she be able to regurgitate her experience, to put it somehow outside of herself, so that someone else might share in its burden. I was of course happy to bear witness, but in this moment, I felt compelled to participate.

"Anne, I want to share something with you, something I have not spoken about very often, but something I want you to know."

"Many years ago, my daughter Lauren was diagnosed with thyroid cancer, my wife Alicia and I sat in the same pre-operative area as you and Steve. Our daughter was set to enter those same mysterious confines of the operating rooms on the third floor of the Milstein Hospital Building. The surgery was not meant to be as long as Bill's, it was expected to take about an hour and a half, not five to six hours, but she needed to be intubated to receive general anesthesia. We were similarly terrified as she disappeared through the green door with the sign, RESTRICTED AREA, OPERATING ROOMS, AUTHORIZED ENTRY ONLY. It is a surreal experience for a parent to watch their child disappear, believe me I know exactly how you felt."

"My goodness, I had no idea," Anne said. "Is she alright now? What's happened to her?"

"Yes, she is fine. Her cancer of course was less aggressive than Bill's, but the fear of its returning is never far."

Anne put her hand on my back and something between us had shifted. No longer was I doctor and she parent, we were equals: two parents, profoundly terrified for their children.

She continued.

"Bill was finally out of surgery and he had survived. My initial relief gave way to a greater need, and I remember thinking, *Okay, now I want more. I want good news.*"

Anne remembered thinking, *My prayers were answered.* "When Dr. Klein returned, he had an enormous smile on his face. He was pleased with the results of the surgery; all of the tumors had been removed and the remaining lymph nodes had been similarly excised. He told us he'd had to remove the lower and middle lobes of Bill's right lung, but that the top lobe had been left intact.

"'Recovery will be difficult,' Dr. Klein told us. 'He will be in the ICU for several days and he will have some pain, but we will load him up with analgesics and we need to be certain he doesn't get pneumonia or an infection. All in all, this is a great day for Bill and for you.'

"'Dr. Klein,' I said, 'May I give you a hug?'

"The post-op recovery was rough, as you might imagine. I think you were on service, I recall seeing you, so you know just how difficult it was. Finally, slowly, day by day, Bill started to improve; drains were removed, pain subsided, nausea and vomiting lessened, fever dissipated. Discharge and home were in sight at last. But, just as we thought we would be leaving the hospital Dr. Blade Gender told us that because recovery was longer than expected she was recommending that we resume the next cycle of chemotherapy as soon as Bill was up to it. This meant that after a mere two weeks of recovering from surgery, Bill would have to stay another five to six days for another round of chemo before he would be able to come home. This was brutal. We were all devasted. But what choice did we have? Frankly none.

"Wait there is more: a new treatment. Dr. Blade Gender wanted Bill to receive radiation therapy and a change in chemotherapy would be needed. She told us that the six-drug regimen he has been receiving could not be given during radiation, thus he would have to switch to an aggressive, two-drug regimen to enhance the positive effects of radiation while simultaneously reducing the potential negative side effects. The new drug protocol would be administered as an outpatient, which meant no more hospital stays for chemotherapy. The radiation treatments would be administered Monday through Friday for seven weeks, a total of 33 encounters. Remarkably, he tolerated the irradiation better than anyone expected. Bill never ceased to surprise. He insisted on attending school. He set his alarm for 6:30, showered and dressed quickly, ate a bowl of oatmeal, grabbed his knapsack, and got ready to go to school. It was his first day at Indian Hills High School in more than five months. He got out of the car with a backpack and a smile and off he went. I sat in the car after he entered the building, overwhelmed by how much I love him and how incredibly proud I am of him."

"I picked him up every day at the school, drove across the GW Bridge to Columbia for his treatment and then drove home during rush hour. He had so much to talk about, so much to tell me about his day. He talked about school all the way to the hospital and all the way home. I was giddy, filled with an incredible sense of joy. He was exhausted and his body was hurting, but he was happy.

"Steve and I talked to each other about our concerns, but we never discussed them with Bill. We watched him get stronger, return to school, spend time with friends, sleep in his own bed, and be with his family. He even found the time to apply to the University of Pennsylvania as an early decision applicant. For now, we had much to celebrate and be thankful for. Maya Angelou wrote, 'Hope and fear cannot reside in the same place. Invite one to stay.' We remind ourselves every day that we must choose hope."

"But, the truth was, Bill was still sick, vulnerable to this disease. Just before Thanksgiving Bill had another round of surveillance CT scans of his chest and abdomen. We expected a good report. However, when we met with Jacki and Hanna the next day we knew immediately something was wrong.

"They telegraphed the news in the eyes and facial expression; they looked despondent.

"'It's bad isn't it,' I cried.

"'Yes.'

"Bill's cancer had recurred with vengeance; he had disease throughout his chest and abdomen. We were devasted. He had months of hell on earth and for what, for this, his cancer was back and more widespread than when he was first diagnosed. We had to tell Bill that the chemotherapy, surgery, and radiation did not control his cancer, the NUT midline carcinoma. The uphill battle suddenly headed downward."

Eternal Peace

The most terrifying words a parent can hear are, "Your child has cancer." Hearing those words and knowing that you, as a parent, are helpless, utterly incapable of protecting your child in the way that nature has biologically programmed, is not simply devastating, it is unmooring, unnatural, it is not right, and yet, there is nothing you can do. If you can, imagine this feeling, and then, try to magnify it by a factor of 10, 100, or a 1,000, no, perhaps infinity. That is the depth of despair, shock, and fear a parent experiences in hearing, "Your cancer is back, it has recurred."

I have spoken these words far too often, to families, teenagers, and young adults. It never gets easy, it gets harder and harder. My years of experience and knowledge have provided me a window to the future. When confronted with a new patient at the time of diagnosis, I have an intuitive sense of who will survive and be cured, and who will not. Those patients with acute leukemia, lymphoma, Hodgkin's disease, and Wilms' tumor, regardless how sick at presentation have a high likelihood of survival; whereas children and adolescents with brain tumors, poor prognosis and metastatic solid tumors, and patients similar to Bill Oliver with rare, impossible to treat cancers have little chance of survival.

I often review the list of active on-therapy patients cared for on our oncology service at Columbia, and silently reflect upon who will live and who will die. This is not a complicated mathematic formulation that requires a PhD in computational science, but rather the state of the art of my subspecialty, child and adolescent oncology in 2020. Overall significant, outstanding results are recorded for some diseases, but with respect to others the prognosis has not changed in my 40 years in practice. It will be up to the next generation to unravel these mysteries and discover novel, innovative yet to be determined treatments as the standard chemotherapy, surgery, and radiation have not moved the needle.

As a cancer patient and the father of a cancer survivor, I am terrified every time I go to my oncologist, or when Lauren visits her doctor for a check-up and scans. The dread of recurrence and constant trepidation is like the Sword of Damocles syndrome, waiting for news and expecting it to be bad, as if your head is going to be chopped off with one mighty swing of the executioner's blade. Cancer patients, myself included, often experience another phenomenon wherein every new ache, pain, low grade fever, or upset stomach signifies a relapse and one cannot help but think, *Holy shit, this must be my cancer.*

The cancer patient's inescapable hypochondriacal attitude and approach to their illness is consuming, perhaps not daily or weekly, but is always present, waiting just below the surface. It takes decades to truly relax, and find acceptance, to be able to identify oneself as a true cancer "survivor," one that no longer fears the Sword of Damocles.

––––––––––––

Anne and Steve wanted to give Bill the news at home, surrounded by his family and belongings, not at the sterile and necessarily uncomforting hospital. Anne later recounted to me that after a dinner of fried chicken and mashed potatoes from the Market Basket, one of Bill's favorite haunts, everyone headed down to the family room to talk.

"'Bill, we have to tell you something.'"

Bill knew immediately what Anne had to tell him. He knew that his cancer had returned and that it was incurable.

"'I knew all along that my case was hopeless. But what can I do? Nothing.'"

Anne's heart broke. This boy, so resigned, so accepting of his wretched fate, this boy was not the Bill she knew, the Bill who went to every track meet and ran his heart out, who studied as hard as possible with the dream of making it to Penn. Anne wanted to remind him of these things, to remind him of who he was, in his heart, at his core, her little boy, but she found herself unable to speak.

"'Bill, we still have to fight,' Steve said.

"'No, we don't Dad, I'm tired. I hate the hospital. I hate being sick all the time. I'm finished. I'm 18 and I can make my own decisions. No more.'"

Strangely, and uncharacteristically for her, Anne was calm, even resigned. She shared with me that Bill had told Hanna, one of his doctors, his friend and confidant that he really did not want treatment in the first place. He believed his NUT midline carcinoma was fatal and that he would die anyway. He allowed the chemotherapy, surgery, and radiation for only one reason, so his parents could believe they did all they could. He had put his parents' desires and wishes above his own.

But acquiescence was finished. Bill needed to assert his own needs and take control of whatever time he had left. He told Steve, Paul, Elizabeth, and Anne, "'I'm done with this shit. I want to go to school as long as I can, be with my friends and Grace, sleep in my own bed. I want to eat Mom's cooking. It's over, I'm going to die, I don't like it, but I accept it. There's nothing I can do to stop this from happening, nothing.'"

Bill got up and went to his room. Anne heard him on his cell phone talking to his girlfriend, Grace. She knocked on his door, "'Honey may I come in?'

"'Of course, Mom, just give me a minute to say goodbye to Grace.'"

Anne waited, unsure of what she would say when she went back in. She wanted to give him his privacy, to allow him to feel the entirety of what he needed to feel, to give him some modicum of control over a situation where control no longer existed. After a few moments that nevertheless felt like an eternity, she opened the door to his bedroom.

Moving toward Bill, she reached out, and soon they were hugging one another uncontrollably, as if holding on would keep him from slipping away. They were both crying.

"'Mom,' Bill said. 'I'm so scared. Why is this happening to me? What did I ever do to deserve this? What the *fuck*!'

"'Honey, I have no answers for you, I wish I did. I pray every day and night that this is a bad dream, but it isn't. I have only one thing to ask, one small favor to ask for Dad and me please. Let's speak to Dr. Blade Gender and see what she has to tell us. Let's not make any decisions until we speak to her. What do you say? Please, honey let's speak to her.'

"'Let me think about it, Mom. I just want to go to sleep, okay?'"

Anne nodded.

"'I love you, Bill. I'm so sorry this happened to you. I am angry at God for letting this happen. You are my life. I understand your desire to rest and be at peace, but let's please speak to the doctor tomorrow, promise me?'

"'Let's discuss in the morning, Mom. I'm too tired to think right now.'"

Anne was tired too. So was Steve. Not sleepy tired, but zombie-like, the worn down, exhaustion of the waking dead. Though of course, the irony was not lost on Anne that she was still very much alive. Had she been able to exchange this exhaustion for her son's illness, she would have in a heartbeat. But, wishful thinking is a luxury extended only to those who are well, not to those dealing with terminal cancer in an 18-year-old's body.

The daily grind had become a torture of its own. Getting through each day was a struggle. Each day required an enormous expenditure of energy and adrenaline, and often Anne felt that she simply would not make it. Staying on top of medicine and injections that had to be administered at precise times throughout the day and night, preparing the house for everything the family needed, managing Bill's pain and nausea, cleaning up vomit, cleaning and changing dressings, making Bill comfortable, making sure he was eating, drinking and brushing his teeth . . . and of course, keeping his spirits up. That was the hardest part.

The Monday after Thanksgiving, Bill relented and Bill, Steve, and Anne returned to the hospital to speak with Jacki Blade Gender. There was no longer any reason to shield Bill from the ugly, wrenching truth. Jacki, although compassionate, was direct and truthful. Addressing Bill, she told him his cancer had recurred and appeared to be spreading rapidly throughout his chest and abdomen. She told Bill that she was not certain there was anything that would halt the aggressive nature of his disease, that though she had searched the medical literature and spoken to several doctors at Columbia and other institutions, she'd concluded there was nothing that could effectively control this horrific cancer. But, she told him that gemcitabine and paclitaxel, a new two-drug combination might slow the progression and mitigate pain.

"'We can administer these drugs in the clinic and keep you out of the hospital,' she told him. 'Christmas at home is a priority.'

"'No more,' Bill told her. 'Especially if it has little hope of working. I'm just so tired. I don't want to be nauseous or vomiting anymore. I'd rather deal with the cancer and pain and be at home with my family and friends and maybe even go to school. But I'll talk it over with Mom and Dad and get back to you.'"

On Wednesday, Bill was back in clinic to begin the new regimen. Jacki had promised his parents that if the side effects of therapy were unbearable, the chemotherapy would be discontinued. Bill believed her.

The entire faculty, fellows, and staff discuss all problematic cases weekly, so I was aware of Bill's status and knew that his disease had recurred, though I was not his primary physician. I was the attending covering the outpatient clinic on Wednesdays, so when Bill and Anne arrived I greeted them, exchanging our firm handshakes, and asked how Bill was doing. I knew he had applied early decision to the University of Pennsylvania.

I asked them, "Have you heard from U. Penn?"

"No, not yet. I think the decisions go out December 15th, so another week or so."

I have always enjoyed caring for teenagers and young adults significantly more than younger children. The conversation about school, sports, music, and other topics is collegial and helps to fortify the relationship. In addition to treating their cancer, I feel I have an opportunity to influence their future.

With Bill's family, I felt a strong bond of trust. I was invested in their well-being, and I felt that I was in a position to help, even beyond whatever medical expertise I might be able to lend. In particular, I always welcome the opportunity to discuss colleges with patients, discussing the virtues of big schools versus small schools, city versus rural, pre-med courses versus business and law. It's an often-welcome distraction for me, a chance to learn from them, and a bonding experience that takes us all beyond the hospital's walls.

Anne had told me several weeks before Bill's renewed therapy, of his interest in the University of Pennsylvania. I encouraged him to apply, even knowing that his cancer had recurred. It seemed to be an important experience psycho-emotionally, a way for him to feel, even briefly, that he was just another normal high school student.

He applied early decision. I suspect he knew that even if accepted he would never matriculate, but that did not stop him from pursuing his dream. I told him I had a dear friend who served on the board of trustees at Penn,

and was a major benefactor to the school. I asked his permission to contact
Herb Roberts on his behalf. He accepted the offer with gratitude.

"No promises," I told him. "But let's see if there's anything that he can do."

"Understood."

———————

Herb Roberts is a fascinating guy with a wonderful story of success. He
was raised in Monticello, New York a one-time resort town in the Catskill
Mountains, north of the city. It was the home to the famous Borscht Belt
hotels, the Concord and Grossingers. His father owned a gas station and
convenience store, worked seven days a week, and raised a family of three
boys. Herb was the middle child. He went to the college at the University
of Buffalo, did well and transferred to the Wharton School of Business at
Penn, where he met his wife Kayla, a nursing student.

Herb's first financial services position was as a First Boston/Credit Suisse
investment banker, but a master's degree in business administration from
Harvard, and befriending Barry Gray, were the transformational events
that shaped his professional career. Together, they founded BlackRock in
1988; Barry became CEO and Herb, President. Their successful partnership created a global investment management corporation that today man-
ages more than six trillion dollars in assets.

George Stein, my oldest childhood friend, introduced me to Herb and
Barry when we lived in Tenafly, New Jersey, 25 years ago. But it was Herb
and Kayla, an oncology nurse, that Alicia and I gravitated towards, and
with whom we developed a deep and long-lasting friendship. Herb is a
man of tremendous emotional depth. He is an astute thinker, gregarious,
honest, humble, philanthropic, and has an incredible sense of humor. He
is a natural leader—people seek his advice, both personally and professionally. His colleagues in the financial community revere him, hold him in
highest regard and are eager to follow and please. For all these reasons Herb
was the first and only person I asked to assist me in founding The Hope

& Heroes Children's Cancer Fund, an independent 501(c)(3) charity dedicated to raising money for the pediatric oncology program at Columbia University Medical Center. We asked our mutual friend Paul Angelos, managing director at Kramer Levin Naftalis & Frankel LLP to complete the necessary legal documents and filings, formed a board of directors that included friends, family, and parents of former patients.

Since its inception, Hope & Heroes has raised close to $75 million. The charity provides resources for patient and family needs including rent, utilities, medications, and transportation. It supports new programs like the Center for Integrative Medicine, developmental therapeutics, and the Center for Survivor Wellness. The charity has enabled recruitment and retention of faculty and has raised $2.5 million for each of four endowed chairs. The chief of the division is the Herb and Kayla Roberts Endowed Professor, and upon my retirement there will be two Michael Weiner, MD endowed professorships for key faculty.

Although Herb readily admits that Hope & Heroes is his favorite charity, his philanthropy encompasses the University of Pennsylvania, the United Jewish Appeal, and the American Cancer Society, among many others. Thus, he was the logical person to approach and ask for his support of the early enrollment application of Bill Oliver to his alma mater. I called Herb's office, and his assistant Kathi Vida told me he was in London, but that she would get in touch and ask him to call me as soon as possible. I told Kathi I would send an email as well so he would have an idea about why I needed to speak with him.

Herb its Michael, I hope you are well and safe in London. I have a favor to ask. We have a patient, Bill Oliver, who applied to Penn early decision. He is a senior at Indian Hills High School in Allendale, New Jersey. He is an excellent student; his average is 3.75 and SAT scores are 1440. He plays soccer, but his claim to fame is his prowess as a long-distance runner, he runs a four minute and fifteen second mile and is being heavily recruited to run track and cross country in college. It is his dream to go to the University of Pennsylvania and he applied early decision. But, Herb, one more thing he has a fatal, rare, tumor that has recurred and he has only weeks to live, he will never matriculate, he will never attend college, will never be a member of the freshman class and he will never run in the Penn Relays as a member of the host school's team. It is his dream to attend college at Penn. Would you contact your colleagues in Philadelphia tell them about Bill and endorse his acceptance.

I pressed "send."

My cell phone chimed in less than five minutes and the screen indicated Herb Roberts.

"Hey Herb, thanks for calling so quickly."

"Are you kidding, of course I'll do whatever I can for Bill. I'll reach the Dean of Admissions directly. Do me a favor, ask Bill to forward me a copy of his college essays, his board scores, transcript, whatever he has so I can acquaint myself with him as best I can."

"Thanks, man. Will do"

Bill and Anne were still in clinic. Anne was reading the Bergen Record, Bill was dozing, it had been another long day, but he seemed to be tolerating the new concoction without too much toxicity.

I approached mother and son, Bill beneath his favorite blue blanket. I gently touched him on the leg and he awoke. "Bill, I spoke to Herb Roberts and he said he would intercede on your behalf. He asked me to have you send him your transcripts, scores, essay, anything you have so he can know as much about you as possible. I told him about your cancer, but no worries, he will help and do whatever he can on your behalf. He said he would try to speak to the Dean of Admissions directly. I'm going to give you his email address and you can communicate with him directly and send him your stuff. Actually, let me have your email address and I will introduce and connect you to one another."

Bill looked up at me and it was hard to tell if he had sleep or tears in his eyes. "Thank you."

"Good luck, Bill. I hope it helps, remember no promises."

Herb and Bill communicated and actually connected several times. Herb did speak to the head of admissions and was told that Bill's application would certainly be competitive for Penn, however, it would be up to Garrett Hickey, the track coach, to determine whether the name Bill Oliver appeared on his list of student-athlete applicants. The head coach of each varsity intercollegiate sport prepared a list of recruited student-athletes that met Penn's academic standards and who they wanted on their respective teams. Herb learned that Coach Hickey in any other circumstance would have been beyond thrilled to have a mile runner of Bill's potential on his squad representing the University of Pennsylvania, but Bill's situation was not normal; the coach knew of Bill's cancer and that he would never run the mile in Franklin Field. Thus, no guarantees.

The gemcitabine and paclitaxel did not slow down the progression of the NUT midline carcinoma. Bill was admitted for management of pain, nausea, and vomiting, and to establish hospice care with the Butterflies team. In general, he was as well as could be expected at home, and was coming to the clinic twice a week for transfusions, medication adjustments, hydration, etc., whatever he needed. Anne and I spoke regularly, we both found it of great value, but for different reasons. She needed to keep her son alive as long as possible, and sharing her memories and thoughts with me was an important part of her process. I, on the other hand, wanted to hear first-hand what it was like to have a child with terminal cancer, every detail, every reflection, every emotion, the highs, the lows and Anne was the perfect vehicle, a wonderfully honest, passionate storyteller.

Mid-December, less than two cold weeks until Christmas. Bill was holding his own, stable, comfortable and thrilled to be at home. He was taking the Vorinostat, but knew it was a smoke screen, with virtually no possibility of having a meaningful effect and even less chance of prolonging his life. Nevertheless, he promised his parents that he would take the drug so long as the toxicity was tolerable and he did not need to stay in the hospital.

Bill was anxious to tell me the news, as he had received notification regarding his early decision application to Penn. I closed my eyes momentarily and said a brief silent prayer, "Please let this extraordinary young man have the joy of acceptance and good news."

"Hey, Dr. Weiner," we shook hands, his grip was strong.

"Good morning, Bill."

"I got wait-listed."

"Really? Wait-listed?"

His eyes told the story, he was more than disappointed.

I was outraged. I tried hard to hide my anger. What the hell were they thinking? They knew damn well that he would never matriculate. Herb Roberts had certainly informed the admissions office of Bill's terminal cancer, that he would not survive. I was reasonably certain that his high school track coach and his guidance counselor at Indian Hills High School had likewise informed the admissions committee of Bill's plight, how could they not? And yet those assholes did not see clear to make the wish of a dying student come true and accept him? No, they wait-listed him. What were they thinking? Excuse me, but screw you University of Pennsylvania.

The Oliver family spent their last Christmas together at home surrounded by family and friends. Neighbors decorated their home, inside and out, with colorful lights and ornaments. It was a joyful time, good food, laughter, good cheer, and exchanging presents. Bill was alright, ate what he could, slept in his own bed, and spent time with Grace. She was wonderful to him, they held hands, hugged each other often, and talked all night long. I learned that when she was about five years old, Grace and her family were friendly with a family called the Matthews. Matt Mathews, her play-mate and kindergarten school buddy, had a brain tumor and died. I often wonder what she remembers of Matt. How tragic for her to experience the loss of not one, but two close friends. Life is not fair. Not fair to Bill, to his brother Paul and sister Elizabeth, to Steve and to Anne, and not fair to Grace.

With the dawn of the new year, Bill's family visited the hospital less. Bill stopped taking the chemotherapy and Anne and Steve supported his deci-sion. Their visits to the hospital became less frequent, though they spoke with Jacki Blade Gender and Hanna frequently by phone and email. Bill spent more time in his room or on the couch in the family room asleep, resting peacefully, waiting for the end.

Bill welcomed the warmth of the family room, it was open to the kitchen and on the far wall there was a fireplace, above it a large 52-inch Samsung. The family kept a fire burning in the hearth for warmth. The couch was large and comfortable, big enough to accommodate Bill's 6-foot, 2-inch frame. It was soft, but not too soft, and he liked resting wrapped in two large wool comforters. Best of all, Anne could keep a covert eye on him from the kitchen, and Bill seemed to glean some relief in knowing she was nearby.

Anne reported the Butterflies nurses to be fantastic. She said that they had become part of the family, that they spent endless hours in the Oliver's home, ensuring that Bill was comfortable and without pain. Anne wel-comed them into their home, particularly Laura and Karen, two wonderful nurses who put Bill and the entire family at ease. They were hardworking, kind, and unobtrusive, and having them around gave Anne peace of mind. With 16 hours of daily coverage, including Saturday and Sunday, the Ol-ivers spent many hours with the Butterflies nurses, drinking coffee and eating snacks from the Market Basket at the kitchen table.

Bill's friends, including Grace, were back at school after the winter holiday break. Steve went back to work at his office and the house was quiet. Bill was calm and pain free, but spoke very little. Anne tried to engage him in conversation, but he was lethargic from the analgesic narcotics needed to control his pain. It is hard work getting ready to die. Anne often tried to snuggle up to Bill on the couch, to hold him, to caress him, and kiss him, her beautiful son.

In a journal she kept she wrote, *I love him so much and to say my heart is broken with sorrow is inadequate. How does a mother watch her son slowly die, closer each day to the end? I was speechless and my sadness was indescribable.*

Toward the end of January, the family noticed that Bill's breathing became labored. They spoke to Jacki and asked if they should bring him back to the hospital, but decided against making the trip, agreeing that if he began to struggle to breathe, the nurses would increase the morphine intravenously to mitigate against the air hunger and feeling of suffocation. Bill was cognizant of what was happening to him, and realized he had two important tasks that must be completed. He called his mother to his side.

"'Mom it's Grace's 18th birthday on February 1st. Help me to buy her a special present.'"

Shopping online they found a beautiful piece of jewelry made in Israel. Bill selected the bracelet, a set of two hammered, silver bangles joined together by a tiny hammered, copper heart. On one of the bangles, the word "love" was hammered.

Bill's second task was harder. At 18 years old, Bill would have to say goodbye to life, to his future, and to his mother.

"'Mom,' he said. 'I need to tell you something. I'm really sick, I'm tired, and I need to go to a better place. I'm ready to die, Mom. I love you and Dad so much, but I can't do this anymore, please tell me it is alright not to fight anymore, please tell me it is okay for me to go, I want to die. I'm so sorry, Mom.'

"'I love you, Bill.'"

Anne and Bill began to cry. Laura, the Butterflies nurse, was crying as well.

"'Bill, thank you. Thank you for being you, thank you for fighting to survive. My darling, boy you have my permission to die.'

"'Thank you, Mom.'"

———————

Bill died on January 25th.

Grace's gift arrived from Israel and Anne gave it to her at his wake.

After the funeral I spoke to Anne. She told me how beautiful the ceremony had been, about the tremendous outpouring of love and respect from all who had known Bill. She told me about her unimaginable grief and her grief about the future that would never be. We will never know what path Bill would have taken or how far he would have gone or what he could have achieved. We know that he had the potential for greatness and happiness and that his future was stolen from him.

Anne recounted her sadness and told me, "We will not get to see him go to his senior prom with Grace. He will not graduate from high school. There will be no last summer before college. He will not go to the University of Pennsylvania. We will never know who he would become and how he would impact the world around him. We will never know if he and Grace would have married. He is dead. He will never have children. They will never exist. His life and his lineage are over."

Some months after Bill's death Anne and I spoke again and it was clear to me that her grief had not subsided, nowhere close. She explained that there are just so many layers of pain and grief. That she missed him desperately and constantly with a sense of longing that will never go away.

"My son is never coming back."

She told me that she missed seeing his face, his sea of freckles and his beautiful green eyes, his tall body coming down the hallway from his room, and thinking he may have grown a little bit more since yesterday. She missed his jokes and their conversations, hearing his thoughts and opinions—learning from him. She missed hugging him and feeling his trim body wrapped in her arms with her face into the crook of his neck. She misses the smell of his deodorant and cologne, his sweet, gentle kisses, his voice, and his infectious laugh. She missed hearing him say, "I love you." She missed his incredible smile and the way it filled her with happiness. She missed the joy and pride he brought her every single day. She missed seeing Bill in his kitchen chair. "He doesn't sit there anymore and his chair is empty now," she said, "Much like my heart."

Everyone Said Not to Worry

My family, like most, has been touched by cancer. Cancer is ubiquitous; it is everywhere. It lurks in the shadows; it is just around the corner, down the street. It is, in the words of Siddhartha Mukherjee, "The Emperor of All Maladies."

When my daughter Lauren was 24 years old, she went to see Kim Kindle, an internist who was on the faculty at Columbia University Medical Center. Her office was located at 800 Fifth Avenue, on the fourth floor, a very tony address on 61st in Manhattan. Lauren was feeling well; her visit was for an annual check-up. Kim, as is her custom, did a complete history, physical examination, and blood work. She routinely spends an hour and a half with each new patient, and although she doesn't accept insurance and charges $1,500 for a new visit, her time and expertise are well worth it.

Case in point, at the conclusion of each visit, it is her routine to review all the findings with her patient. At the end of Lauren's visit, she told her that during the exam, she'd felt a small nodule on her thyroid gland, an organ in the neck that overlies the throat. Now, I have examined the thyroid thousands of times and only once have I ever felt something unusual. Kim reassured Lauren that this is quite common and the vast majority—more than 95 percent—of such nodules are benign. However, she recommended an ultrasound of Lauren's neck in order to visualize the lump.

Fortunately, I was able to make a phone call and get the sonogram of the thyroid done the same day; just one benefit of working at Columbia Presbyterian for as long as I had. The thyroid ultrasound confirmed the presence of the nodule, a fine needle aspirate to take a small sample of the nodule for testing would be next.

Again, the radiologist indicated that it looked benign on the scan. "So please don't be concerned."

The next day, a bright, cold afternoon in late January, I accompanied Lauren to the radiology department on the third floor of the Milstein Hospital building, part of Columbia Presbyterian's sprawling campus on the Upper West Side. Lauren, usually anxious, seemed stoic and calm, taciturn and ready to have the procedure behind her. Dr. Cheryl Mazur-Gordon, a young-ish radiologist, took Lauren into the examination room. The room was small, no more than 100 square feet, with bare walls and low lighting to allow the doctor and technician to better view the sonogram pictures on the screen. An exam table stood in the middle of the room for the patient, and a stool sat in front of the monitor for the doctor.

Dr. Mazur-Gordon, who many years later would become my friend at the hospital, asked Lauren to remove her shirt, don a hospital gown, and lie down on the examination table. She cleaned and prepped her neck with betadine and placed a sterile cover over the ultrasound probe. She began the procedure, scanned the thyroid, localized the nodule, and marked the spot on the surface of Lauren's neck. Next, she took a small 25-gauge needle affixed to a syringe and carefully entered the gland at the location of the marker to aspirate the nodule. She then placed the contents on a glass slide and put the slide in a slide-box container. She repeated this process three times. All samples were appropriately labeled. All told, the procedure took about 10 or 15 minutes.

Fifteen minutes, I thought. *A mere 15 minutes of clinical procedure could forever alter the course of my life and my daughter's.*

"The majority of these nodules are benign," Dr. Mazur-Gordon assured Lauren again as we prepared to leave. "We'll know for certain in a few days.

It takes about two to three days for the results to become available, and the pathologist will notify Dr. Kindle with the results."

———————————

We were silent as we walked to the physician's parking lot on 165th Street, got into my car, and drove to our home in Tenafly, just north of the George Washington Bridge in New Jersey. After a long while, Lauren turned to me, her stoic resolve quickly dissolving. "Dad," she said. "Do you think I have cancer?" Her voice faltered. "I'm scared."

Frankly, I was scared, too. The doctors' reassurances had given me little solace. All too often, I have treated patients whose illnesses contradicted statistics. Medicine is not exact, and diagnoses are more guidelines than roadmaps. Could my little girl have cancer?

Waiting was the hard part. As the hours turned to days, I thought about Lauren.

I thought about the day she'd been born. Alicia had woken up early, feeling contractions every two to three minutes, and had called Karl Edwards, her obstetrician. He told us to meet him at the Harkness Pavilion in the early afternoon and instructed us to page him when we arrived. Alicia was tired, and more than a little bit anxious. Her first pregnancy had ended in a miscarriage, so while she was certainly excited to give birth to our healthy little girl, her excitement was tinged with apprehension. I knew that I could do little to assuage her anxiety. It was a gorgeous day in early May, the perfect time of year for a run outside.

"Honey," I said. "Do you mind if I go for a quick run in Central Park? Will you be okay without me?"

"Yes," she replied, very independent. "But I still want to take a ride to the Baby Outlet on Queens Boulevard before we go to the hospital. I want to buy that pale pink comforter for Lauren."

"You're kidding," I said. "You're about to give birth, and you want to go to Queens? Why don't you just relax?"

"I'll be fine." By the look on her face, I could tell that this was an argument not worth pursuing.

I threw on a pair of shorts and a tee shirt, laced up my blue Nikes, and jogged to the park, a short block away from our apartment on the corner of 87th and Madison Avenue. I ran a leisurely five-mile loop, thinking about all that was to come. I had faith that the delivery would be smooth, but still, I would be lying if I said that I didn't have some apprehensions. Alicia's pregnancy had been uneventful; she felt well throughout. She had an amniocentesis during her second trimester and the results indicated nothing unusual or worrisome. Everything indicated that, within hours, our first child, a healthy baby girl would be born.

Back at home, Alicia's resolve was intact, so we loaded up the car with everything we'd need at the hospital and made a pit stop in Queens before heading to the hospital. Her maternity bag included a white nightgown and matching robe from Bloomingdales, slippers, her favorite pillow, recent copies of Vogue and Bazaar magazines, her insurance card, a notebook and pen, and, of course, the new pink and white comforter for the baby.

We arrived at the hospital at 3 p.m. and paged Dr. Edwards. He assured us that Alicia was hours away from delivery and admitted her to a private room on Harkness 11, the labor and delivery floor, where we waited for six hours with no visible progress. Dr. Edwards ordered pelvic x-rays and concluded that Alicia would need a caesarian section. We were both relieved; the contractions were uncomfortable, her cervix was not dilated sufficiently, and labor was not progressing. We knew that babies born by C-section are unscathed—no forceps, no squeezing through the birth canal.

Alicia told Dr. Edwards, "No problem, let's do it now, its baby time."

The amniocentesis performed several months earlier indicated we were going to have a girl, we had already picked a name that began with L in memory of my grandfather, Laurence. We'd chosen the name Lauren, goddess of wisdom, from a book of French names that we'd purchased on a earlier trip to Paris.

Lauren was born at 1 a.m. on May 6, 1979. My goodness, she was beautiful. A full head of dark hair, green eyes, full cheeks, perfect features, weighing 7 pounds, 11 ounces. She was perfect.

Joyful and healthy, she walked and talked and virtually toilet-trained herself. I recall one Christmas season when she was about three years old, she was running a temperature just over 104 degrees. Delirious, she turned to me and said, "The Christian people think Jesus is the son of God, but the Jewish people think he is a lawyer."

Lauren learned to figure skate when she was five, and it was often my responsibility to chaperone. Many winter Saturday and Sunday mornings were spent at Wohlman Rink at the southern end of Central Park with the Plaza Hotel in the background, as Lauren twirled around on the ice. Carrie French, a resident, fellow, and friend from my Mt. Sinai days joined us when she was able; Carrie, a former Olympic figure skater, enjoyed skating with Lauren and Wohlman Rink is an idyllic spot. These mornings were our time together, father and daughter, and I felt proud watching my graceful skater gliding and spinning across the ice. While the Zamboni cleaned and scraped the surface between sessions, we'd drink hot chocolate and eat glazed donuts.

Lauren went to an all-girls performing arts summer camp, Belvoir Terrace, in Lenox, Massachusetts with her cousins Brooke and Rose Klein. The camp owners, Edna Goldberg and her daughter, Nancy, insisted upon meeting the prospective campers in their New York City apartment on Central Park West for an interview and mini performance. Lauren played the piano. She sat at the baby grand keyboard, and Nancy, expecting to hear a Mozart piano concerto, was treated to "Chopsticks." We were all hysterical. She played it flawlessly.

And now my little doll was facing possible—no, probable—cancer.

We waited.

Pathologists have a difficult job. Very few patients recognize the pressure that pathologists often experience. They are the doctors locked away in a remote part of the hospital, whom all other physicians rely upon to provide answers, and of course, no question is more important than, *Does my patient have cancer?*

In order to answer that question, the pathologist must first take the biopsy samples, which the surgeon placed in either a bottle of Bouin's solution or on a gauze soaked with normal saline, and embed the material in paraffin or wax and wait for it to harden. When the biopsy sample has hardened, they cut the paraffin blocks into ultra-thin tissue with a microtome, which they then place on a slide. The slides are stained with special stains and set aside to dry, and then are ready for interpretation.

The process of slide preparation, review, and diagnosis is repeated hundreds of times each day. Biopsy samples arrive in the Department of Pathology, located in the Vanderbilt Clinic on the 14th through the 16th floors, from not only the operating rooms, but also from the endoscopy suites, interventional radiology, and procedure rooms. Every doctor and every patient want quick results, however, an important lesson and philosophy that must be practiced every single day is 'never rush the pathologist.' Better to be patient and allow them to do their work properly than to rush them and make a mistake.

Their results must be accurate 100 percent of the time—no questions asked.

And so, we waited.

Lauren was certain that the biopsy was going to be positive, and honestly, so did I. Alicia, on the other hand, refused to even allow the thought of possible cancer to enter her mind. Her attitude was that if we would have to deal with it, we would know soon enough, so she did not allow speculation to alter her daily routine.

Lauren and I both tried hard not to Google thyroid cancer, to no avail. It was our constant preoccupation, but a solitary one, as neither of us wanted to admit it to the other. One day became two; two days became three; we were all painfully aware that the weekend was fast approaching. If we didn't hear on Friday we would have to wait until Monday, an additional two days that would seem like an eternity.

Technically speaking, I should not use my network at the hospital to ascertain medical information on a patient not in my care, even if that patient was my daughter. It was morally dubious, but I simply could not wait any longer. I cracked.

I called a friend, Mohammad Bachir, in pathology to see if he could find any information on the needle biopsy performed several days earlier. Hesitant at first, he soon acquiesced when I explained that the sample in question was my daughter's. He called me back within minutes.

"Michael," he said, and I could hear it in his voice. "The biopsy shows papillary thyroid cancer. I'm so sorry, Michael. The final has been signed out, and Kim Kindle has been notified."

My heart sank. Throughout my long career as a pediatric oncologist, I have delivered bad news to thousands of patients and families, but to be on the other side of the desk—to be on the receiving end of that short, devastating sentence—is a different thing entirely.

My child has cancer. The words would not sink in.

Lauren was at her desk on the 30th floor of the BlackRock headquarters on East 52nd Street when the call came from Kim Kindle. BlackRock, one of the largest money managers of fixed income products in the world was founded by Barry Gray and Herb Roberts about 25 years ago. She was a VP in the alternative products section of the company and was a member of the team that specialized in managing real estate assets. George Stein, one of my oldest and dearest friends, introduced me to Barry and Herb, and although they were inseparable business partners, they could not have

been more different. Barry was aloof, close-mouthed, and rather conde-
scending, whereas Herb was gregarious, welcoming, sincere, and honest;
he has become a close friend. Despite his enormous success and wealth, he
is grounded, philanthropic, never forgets a holiday or special occasion, and
always, 100 percent of the time, puts his wife, Kayla, and family first. Together, Herb and I founded the Hope & Heroes Children's Cancer Fund,
an independent 501(c)(3) in 1998. At BlackRock, he is beloved and revered and is a secretive godfather to Lauren at work.

Lauren told me that when she saw Dr. Kindle's name on her iPhone, she
was petrified and did not want to pick up. Though she said that she had
been expecting it, she could not bring herself to hear the words spoken out
loud, making it real. Undoubtedly, she was shaking like a leaf.

Kim spoke very matter-of-factly and without emotion as she told Lauren,
"The biopsy shows that you have papillary thyroid cancer, the most common type of thyroid cancer in young women. You'll need some tests, scans,
and probably surgery, but on the positive side, this is treatable. You should
expect a full recovery. I have already called the office of Dr. Tom James, he
is an expert and will take excellent care of you. You are in good hands."

Lauren hung up the phone, her head spinning, her heart pounding. I'd
been watching my phone closely, expecting her call. I picked up on the
first ring.

"Dad, I have cancer," she gasped. "I'm scared. Am I going to die? I need
to come home to Tenafly—now. I can't be alone this weekend. I need you
and Mom. Can I come meet you? I need to see you." It was difficult to
make out what she was saying. Her breath was hard and heavy, and she was
starting to cry. "I'm going to leave my office now and take a cab to the hospital, wait for me, okay? I knew it. I just knew it. I knew this was going to
happen. What am I going to do? Am I going to be all right? I can't believe
this is happening to me."

I took a deep breath, hoping to slow us both down—an impossible goal.

"Yes, sweetheart, of course you can come meet me," I said, doing my best impression of a calm figure of authority. "You are not going to die. You are going to be just fine. We are going to make sure that you get the absolute best treatment possible, and we are going to beat this thing. You'll live a long, happy life, honey, I promise."

We were both weak and in disbelief.

"Okay, Dad," Lauren said, her voice small. I thought about my little girl, spinning across the ice. "I'm leaving now; I'll see you soon."

I called Evan Cole. He and his wife, Eleanor, had been close friends of ours since we'd first met in 1977. Evan is the Chair of the Department of Surgery at Columbia Presbyterian. He went to Columbia University undergrad and to medical school at Physicians and Surgeons. In his day, he was considered one of the best cardiac surgeons in the country; in 1984, he led the Columbia Presbyterian team that performed the first ever successful heart transplant on a child. It was because of Evan that I returned to Columbia in 1996 to become the Director of Pediatric Oncology. He knew everyone at the medical center.

"Evan, Lauren was just diagnosed with papillary thyroid cancer, and her internist wants her to see Tom James. Do you know him?"

"Yes, he is excellent—really knows his stuff. He is a bit stiff, old school, and conservative, but really solid clinically. He is a good choice for Lauren. She will be okay."

Evan and Eleanor had known Lauren her entire life. In fact, Eleanor, an anesthesiologist, was in the delivery room and administered the epidural anesthetic to Alicia when Lauren was born. Our families have remained intertwined ever since.

I met Lauren on the corner of 165th Street and Fort Washington Avenue. I had a decision to make. Should I be her father or her doctor? I chose the former; however, I recognized that she was analytical and needed information to help her process her future. I was prepared to share with her how I really felt—crestfallen and crushed—but I was also prepared to provide her with whatever she needed: information, understanding, and advice as to how to accept her new reality in order to face an uncertain future. The hospital was full of excellent, competent, caring physicians, but my daughter had only one father. When she approached, I immediately engulfed her in a big bear hug as she wiped away the tears.

"I'm terrified, Dad," she mumbled into my chest.

"Cancer is terrifying, sweetheart," I said. "I'm scared too. But I promise, we'll do whatever it takes to make you well."

Lauren was much closer to Alicia than to me; they spoke every day about whatever it is that mothers and daughters speak about. When Lauren needed me, I knew it was an important question or she needed advice beyond that which Alicia could provide. Our conversations were about job-related issues, money, and, frequently, health issues. We were treading in new territory; me as the father of a child with cancer and Lauren as a cancer patient.

When Lauren and I arrived at our new home—a modern, three-floor townhouse with an elevator on Kensington Court in Tenafly—we found Alicia in the kitchen, preparing pasta primavera for Lauren and a Bolognese sauce for us. Though we'd waited to give her the news in person, Alicia could immediately deduce Lauren's diagnosis from the looks on our faces and the puffiness of her eyes.

Again, Lauren began to cry, "Mom, I'm so scared. I just can't believe this is happening to me. What am I going to do? *What am I going to do?*"

"Shush, my darling, shush. Take a deep breath and try to be calm." Alicia turned off the stove, quickly washed her hands, and embraced Lauren tightly as she wiped away her tears.

My wife and daughter moved to the couch in the living room and held each other tightly. Penelope, our Cavalier King Charles Spaniel, jumped onto the sofa and cuddled next to Lauren, never one to miss an opportunity for human body warmth.

As I watched the two tearfully embrace, I realized sadly that Lauren's understanding of cancer was informed by what I'd shared over the dinner table from my own experiences. The conversations at home were rarely about survivors, usually I talked about children who'd died, since their stories were the ones that stayed with me; the ones I had to keep telling and telling in order to make sense of them. Lauren's frame of reference was distorted. She believed cancer was synonymous with death, though the majority of the patients I cared for survived. My mistake. Nevertheless, she was terrified. She needed to be educated. We both needed to be educated.

As a pediatric oncologist, thyroid cancer was not a disease that I was very familiar with. Its management was the bailiwick of endocrinologists, not cancer specialists, so I was as new to this as my daughter was.

After a few minutes of mother-daughter comfort, Alicia, always the practical one, stood, walked to the kitchen, and finished the dinner preparation. "Come to the table for a bowl of pasta and salad."

We ate quickly and quietly, as Lauren had only one thought on her mind: learn as much about thyroid cancer as possible, fast. As soon as we'd finished, she grabbed her laptop from her bag, opened it on the round table in the living room, and began keying words and phrases into Google, with which we'd quickly develop a close, if slightly codependent, relationship.

We read articles and posts intended for lay-people, but we also reviewed medical literature. Wikipedia, Up-To-Date, and the National Comprehensive Cancer Network (NCCN) guidelines all provided useful information. We printed important articles and made notes to review from others.

We absorbed a great deal of information that weekend, and the more knowledge we acquired, the more relaxed and comfortable we became with the idea that Lauren would be fine. We learned that thyroid cancer was common, especially in young women, and that there were about 50- to 60,000 new cases diagnosed in the United States each year. There are four pathological types: papillary, medullary, follicular, and anaplastic. Lauren had papillary, the most common for young people, and also the one with the highest cure rate, approaching 98 percent long-term survival. We looked into thyroid surgery and fully recognized that an operation would be required in the very near future. We learned about staging, to determine how the cancer spreads either directly to contiguous anatomic structures or through the bloodstream and lymphatic system. We researched treatment with radioactive iodine and thyroid replacement therapy. By the end of the weekend, Lauren was well prepared for her appointment with Dr. James.

Despite what we'd read over the weekend, and despite the strong face I had put on for Lauren, internally, I remained terrified. I knew too well from my own professional experience that there are never guarantees in medicine. Lauren reminded me that Dr. Kindle had told her not to worry, and I felt that she was assuring herself as much as she was me. Dr. Mazur-Gordon had told Lauren not to worry when she'd first found the nodule. She'd told her that most nodules were non-cancerous. Yet here we were. I had personally seen plenty of cases where the odds weren't in the patient's favor, despite what the numbers implied. I was having a hard time finding confidence and faith in our situation.

The Other Side of the Desk

A new cancer diagnosis has a way of testing one's psychic-emotional make-up. Lauren, and our whole family for that matter, were about to find a lot about ourselves, our character, and our inner strength.

Frankly, Lauren's past was not without incident. As a 14-year-old, she flirted with anorexia nervosa. It was about control and rebellion, as that disease so often is. It was deeply unsettling for me to watch my child lose almost 20 percent of her body mass, to weigh less than 100 pounds, and eat four crackers, a scoop of yogurt, and three bites of a banana for an entire day. Fortunately, she was amenable to rapid psychiatric intervention and medical monitoring.

We assembled a terrific team. Dr. Brianna Gardner, her pediatrician, saw Lauren weekly for a weight check and to review her daily food diary. Her therapist, Dr. Lynne Forest, was phenomenal, skillful, caring, compassionate, and available. She had an office on Depeyster Street, a short walk from our family home on Woodhill Road, and she encouraged Lauren to take the five-minute walk to her appointments. She met with Lauren twice a week, and with Alicia and I separately on a regular basis. Alicia was a rock. Despite her full-time job as a principal and executive of J & M Silver, a family-owned and operated fashion jewelry manufacturer, she made our daughter's well-being her first priority.

During the course of the therapy, it became apparent that my relationship with Lauren was problematic, and that I needed to change for my child and for me. I had a quick, explosive temper and tried to control most situations. Frankly, I was a mess. Lynne Forest suggested that I enter psychotherapy to unravel the etiology of my behavior and to learn how to be a better parent, one who exercised restraint, understanding, and support. It was surreal to hear Lauren say, "Dad, you frighten me, and I am afraid that you are going to hurt me."

The message was clear. I began to see a therapist weekly. I saw Dr. Alan Weisenbrot, a senior psychiatrist at Columbia and the New York State Psychiatric Institute, in his private office on East 87th Street. As fate would have it, the office was located on the first floor of the building where our family had lived from 1979 until we moved to Tenafly, New Jersey, in 1993. He occupied a two-room suite: a small, dimly lit waiting room with two chairs, a table, and a lamp; the office itself, was small, the walls had peeling paint, and three artwork posters that announced exhibits at the Metropolitan Museum of Art for Van Gogh and Matisse hung on the walls. There was a desk and a reclining chair for the doctor, a two-person loveseat, and a large comfortable chair. Inevitably, I sat in the chair.

Dr. Weisenbrot helped me to understand the issues I was having and to modify my behavior. Together, we unrecovered past demons. My fallback had always been that my father had a bad temper and that is the explanation for my short fuse. However, I learned that this was unacceptable; my rage was affecting the people I cared about most: my family, Alicia, Lauren, and our son, Eli. The stimulus was about control and having my way. When a situation turned adversely against me, I exploded.

The doctor offered some short-term, simple solutions: count to 10, walk away, don't answer, and engage. He also suggested that I make an audio recording of an outburst so I could appreciate how totally noxious this behavior could be not only to my well-being, but to others as well.

I am certain that he collaborated with Dr. Forest, and together, they helped Lauren emerge from her illness and helped me to not only become a better parent, but a better person as well. Alicia deserves much credit for being the stabilizing influence we needed. Our family healed.

"Dad," Lauren said after another long research session on the couch that weekend. "You are planning to come with me Monday morning to Dr. James, aren't you?"

"Yes, of course. What time is your appointment? I think I'm going to send an email to my friend Hal Short, one of the surgeons at Columbia who does thyroid surgery. Maybe he will be able to see you on Monday after your appointment with Dr. James. Might as well see if he is available, what do you think?"

"Sure."

I emailed Hal, and, quite to my surprise, he called me back immediately. Evan Cole had introduced me to him. Hal also served on the Columbia Doctors board, so we spoke the same language. He was an endocrine surgeon, trained by Dr. Peter Mason, who was one of the foremost thyroid surgeons in the country, and, 40 years ago, was instrumental in describing the surgical technique and approach to a total thyroidectomy. In 1979, Peter operated on me for a right-side hernia repair, and in 2000, Hal performed the same operation on me but on the left side. We had history together.

"Hal, my daughter Lauren was just diagnosed with papillary thyroid cancer. She is seeing James first thing Monday morning. Is there any chance you can see her Monday as well?"

"Sure, I will find the time to see her. I am seeing patients in my office in Irving on Monday morning. I should be able to fit her in. I am going to call my assistant, Barbara, and ask her to give you a call. I should be able to reach her today. Give me your phone number, and I will have her call you."

"Great, but ask her to call Lauren, not me, if that is okay. I will tell her, and she will be expecting the call."

Barbara called about an hour later and told Lauren to come to Dr. Short's office on the eighth floor of the Irving Pavilion when she was finished with

Dr. James. She took personal and demographic information from Lauren and told her to bring her insurance information.

The rest of the weekend was uneventful. Lauren rested and called Callie Posner, a friend from high school and Barnard College, who came over to spend a few hours with her. Lauren later mentioned to us that she had told Callie about her thyroid cancer. Her friend had been very consoling and reassuring; she told Lauren that her mother had been diagnosed with thyroid cancer when she was in her 20s and she had obviously married, had two children, and remained well without any related problems.

Alicia was crazy busy doing whatever Alicia did on the weekends. She did her weekly food shopping at the ShopRite in Englewood, dropped off the dry-cleaning, went to the shoemaker, and still found time to have a manicure and have her hair washed and get a blowout at the local salon.

My sister, Margaret, and my brother-in-law, Gene, introduced me to Alicia. I had been married before for a few years while in medical school in Syracuse. It seemed like the thing to do at the time; many of my classmates were getting married, and the winters were long and cold in Syracuse, New York. So, why not? Wendy and I divorced without much fanfare—we had no real assets, no children, she took the furniture, and I took the car and Maddy, the cocker spaniel. When I think about my first marriage so many years ago, I have one indelible memory that my mother shared with me after the divorce. She recalled that the first time my parents met Wendy and her parents, Howard and Blanche, at their home in Harrisburg, Pennsylvania, to celebrate Passover, she told me father, "Bill, this will never work. Let's take our son and get out of here." Obviously, she was right.

Alicia and I met on April 20th; it was my 30th birthday. We had drinks at the Algonquin Hotel. For our second date, we went to the Parador restaurant on East 34th Street; I still remember to this day that I ordered the most incredible mole chicken. I also recall that, on our third date, I prepared a dinner of sautéed chicken and chicken livers, a recipe from Il Monello, an Upper East Side haunt for Alicia, Margaret, and Gene; it was awesome. The following Saturday, we spent the day together and drove to New Hope,

Pennsylvania, a funky, touristy Delaware River town about two hours west of the city. The day was great, but the night even better. With Maddy on the floor at the foot of Alicia's pullout sofa bed in her studio apartment on Jane Street in the West Village, we made love all night long. I knew at that moment that this was the woman I would spend the rest of my life with; it was simply memorable.

As Lauren and Alicia were settled for the day, I played golf at Alpine Country Club with the Levitt brothers, Barry and Richie, and Sam Saperstein. I really enjoyed golf, I had good friends there, and Alpine was a bastion of comfort for me. The course was a treasure designed by A.W. Tillinghast, one of the most famous golf course architects of the early 20th century. The course is a beautiful, tight, tree-lined layout, with fast undulating greens. It is flat out difficult, but being on the course with friends is as good as it gets. We usually walk, and with caddies carrying the golf bags, I feel as if I am on the 18th fairway at Augusta playing in the Masters with Tiger Woods and Phil Mickelson. Alpine is a gem, and I love being there.

Saturday night, Lauren, Alicia, and I went to Saigon Republic for dinner; the sesame noodles, vegetable dumplings, crispy duck, and lemongrass chicken were delicious, as always. We talked about the day and what Lauren faced Monday morning. She was surprisingly relaxed and prepared to do what she needed to do in order to get well and put thyroid cancer behind her. "Honestly," she said, "I have no choice, do I?"

"Not really, but the immediate path to cure seems clear. My suggestion is to take it one day at a time. You have your appointments on Monday with James and Hal Short, and I think you know that you will at least need surgery. So, let's concentrate on getting through that."

I thought her attitude was great. She most certainly was fearful, but she was primed to accept her diagnosis and do what needed to be done. That night in bed with Saturday Night Live playing on the TV, Alicia and I agreed that Lauren seemed to be in a good place—accepting, realistic, and optimistic. I kissed Alicia tenderly.

"I love you, Alicia."

"I love you too, honey. Goodnight."

We turned off the TV and the lights and fell asleep holding hands.

On Sunday, Eli came home from college, and we went to brunch at Alpine, an over the top buffet that is my favorite excuse to eat as much as possible in a short period of time. My family found going to Alpine a noxious experience. Alicia did not play golf, and Eli had no interest in learning. Lauren interestingly did express interest, and I went so far as to purchase her a starter set of golf clubs, but they remained unused in the storage closet. Like most country clubs, Alpine had a food and beverage minimum, and attending the Sunday buffet helped to reduce that cost. This was my excuse to coerce my family into going to brunch. I enjoyed attending; I was proud of my family, and the hour we spent together was one of the few times we were all together. The children chide me to this day that I seemed like the mayor, greeting everyone, introducing Lauren and Eli to people they had not met previously. They patronized me, Alpine was my haven, not my family's.

Eli is four years younger than Lauren. He stands 6 feet, 3 inches tall (I'm not sure how, as both Alicia and I are of average height). He is a taller version of me, except he has blue eyes whereas mine are brown. As a child and during his early teenage years, Eli was small. He played on the local traveling hockey team from the age of 8 until he was 14 years old. He played defense on the double-A mite, squirt, peewee, and bantam teams. But as a 14-year-old bantam, he weighed under 100 pounds and there were kids on the opposing teams that weighed 50 pounds more and were 6 inches taller. One Saturday as we were driving to a game in Brick Township, New Jersey, he told me, "Dad, I'm getting killed out there, these kids are so big."

That was Eli's last year on hockey skates. He had a tremendous growth spurt when he was 16 that did not stop until he reached his present height. He had no regrets about not playing hockey, though, and while he did play tennis and soccer for The Dwight Englewood School, he did not enjoy sports. He seemed to play because he thought I wanted him to do so, and there may be some truth to that. However, he moved away from sports to considerably more creative pursuits; he wanted to be a filmmaker.

He had just graduated from Columbia University, the absolute worst college for him to attend. The rigid core curriculum at Columbia was nearly his academic demise. However, at the time, the idea of going to an Ivy League school as his other high school friends were matriculating at Harvard and University of Pennsylvania seemed to be the right choice. In addition, as I was a Columbia University faculty member, his tuition was totally paid for as a benefit of my employment.

He should have gone to the Tisch Film School at New York University. He had always been a creative soul; he was more left brain than right, as they say. He looked at the world differently than most and observed things in life that others failed to see. He aspired to be a film writer and director, and I suppose he will one day achieve this lofty goal. It was his single-minded focus to succeed. In addition, he insisted that he would accomplish his personal goals by himself, without any assistance, regardless of how insignificant it might be from me. I always snicker when I see that a new blockbuster film is directed or produced by the offspring of parents who are real estate or financial scions (Roger Scott and Charlie Sharon, cases in point). What would Roger and Charlie achieve had their fathers not been multi-billionaires. Well, maybe they do have talent—who am I to judge?

The remainder of the weekend was uneventful. There wasn't much conversation. We all did our own thing, and Lauren mentally prepared herself for one of the most important days of her life.

Lauren, Evan, and I were up early on Monday morning and drove into the city together. I dropped Evan off at the A Train subway station at the corner of Broadway and 168th Street and then parked the car in the doctor's lot on 165th Street. Lauren went to Dr. James's office on the second floor of the Irving Pavilion, and I went to mine on the seventh floor to leave my attaché case and quickly read through emails to be certain there was nothing urgent that needed my immediate attention. There was not. I told my assistant, Xiomara, that I was going to be with my daughter for a few hours and if she needed me, she was to call my cell phone. I took the back stairs down to the second floor and found Lauren in the waiting room, filling out the obligatory demographic forms, insurance information, and medical history.

The Irving Pavilion, formerly the Atchley Pavilion, is an office building for the clinical practices of Columbia's doctors. The Herbert and Florence Irving Cancer Center occupies renovated space on floors 7 through 14. James's office on the second floor shows more than 50 years of use; it is old and drab with poor lighting and ancient furniture. I sat next to my daughter, who was trying hard to be stoic and accepting of her new reality. Having spent the weekend studying, she had come prepared with a list of questions for her doctor.

Dr. James appeared promptly at 9. He was a tall, gray-haired, distin-guished-looking gentleman in a white coat. He introduced himself to us and suggested that he first spend some time alone with Lauren. He said that he would ask me to join them when he was finished with his history and exam. He explained that it would take about 45 minutes and he would call me when he was ready for discussion.

"Thanks Dr. James, I would appreciate that. My office is just upstairs, and Lauren knows my number."

I stood and watched as he escorted my little girl into his inner sanctum. Lauren seemed so small at that moment. She was a petite 5 feet, 2 inches and had her mother's freckles and a little bump on the bridge of her nose. Her hair was pulled back into a ponytail, and she wore a black sweater and pants and low heels. She looked like a young professional, but instead of going to a business meeting, she was about to learn what her immediate future looked like. We had done our research about thyroid cancer and discussed it on and off throughout the weekend. We both possessed a con-siderable amount of information, so there would be no surprises, or so we hoped.

Dr. James seemed to be the epitome of the outstanding clinicians who made Columbia Presbyterian a paragon of excellent health care for more than a century. Columbia had always been at the forefront of medical observation, patient care, discovery, and innovation, and Tom James fit the mold. His reputation was one of an exemplary doctor and mentor to young physicians-in-training. He had a very paternal manner about him. He seemed to be a good fit for Lauren; I was relieved.

My mobile phone rang at precisely 9:45, as promised.

"Dad, Dr. James said you should come down and join us in his office."

"I'll be right there."

When I arrived downstairs, Dr. James began, "May I call you Michael, and please call me Tom." I accepted willingly. "So, Lauren has a 1 cm nodule in the upper pole of the right lobe of her thyroid. I repeated my own ultrasound, and I do not see anything else of concern. As you know, it's a papillary carcinoma, quite common and very curable. She will need surgery. Lauren tells me that you are going to see Hal Short. He would be my recommendation; he is an excellent surgeon. There are several options for the type of surgery from a lobectomy, to a partial thyroidectomy, to a total thyroidectomy. My suggestion is a total thyroidectomy with a sentinel lymph node sampling."

"Tom, the rationale for a total removal?"

"I fully expect Lauren to be cured of this disease and to live a normal life with a normal life expectancy. She will need thyroid hormone replacement therapy, and it is easier to manage her thyroid function and to follow her after treatment with a total removal. Surgically, for Dr. Short, it is also a more direct and easier operation with less risk of damaging the four parathyroid glands that sit on top of each of the four lobes of the thyroid. It is just cleaner and better."

"Got it. Lauren, do you have questions?"

"No, not now."

"You should let me know the date of the surgery so I can talk to Hal to begin replacement with Synthroid immediately post-op. About four weeks after surgery, we need to do a radioactive iodine thyroid scan to monitor for any aberrant thyroid tissue and to be certain that the surgery was completely ablative."

We stood, shook Dr. James' hand, and left the office. We took the elevator to the eighth floor and walked to Dr. Short's office. We found Barbara, who handed Lauren a clipboard with additional forms to complete. In reality, in 2005, if a patient had consultations with five different physicians despite the fact that there existed an electronic medical record and all the doctors worked at Columbia and the New York Presbyterian Hospital, the records were siloed. Thus, the mandatory paperwork is repeated over and over—how efficient. Barbara told us that Dr. Short was still with another patient, but he was expecting Lauren, "So please make yourself comfortable in the waiting room, I'll tell him you are here."

"Thank you."

The eighth floor was a renovated floor; the unit was well lit and had comfortable furniture and freshly painted pale gray walls. Framed scenes and photographs hung from the walls and there was reading material about the weight loss bariatric program, the pancreatic surgery center, and information about colon cancer screening. There were old *Time* magazines and a couple of ancient *Sports Illustrated* as well, of course. After about 20 minutes, Hal Short appeared. Hal is my height—5 feet, 9 inches—usually wears a suit, white shirt with cufflinks, and usually a colorful Hermès tie. This morning however, he wore a starched white coat with his name printed above the left pocket. He is a stylish guy. He introduced himself to Lauren in his usual soft-spoken manner and asked her to come with him to the exam room. He returned about five minutes later. "Michael, join us."

I had great respect for Hal as a surgeon. He had technical skill at the top of the game. He, too, was a product of the Columbia Presbyterian historical excellence. He was a trained endocrine surgeon with expertise in thyroid, adrenal, and pancreatic surgery. Recently, he had concentrated on surgery for pancreatic cancer and he was one of the few surgeons at Columbia to perform the Whipple operation, a six- to eight-hour procedure to remove the pancreas and surrounding involved lymph nodes and structures. Nevertheless, because of our friendship, he wanted to perform Lauren's thyroid surgery.

"I spoke with Tom James , and he told that there is a 1 cm nodule in the upper right lobe. Honestly, I am not able to feel it on exam. I give a lot of credit to Kim Kindle to have felt it or at least suspected that there might be something there. She is an excellent diagnostician. I also spoke to pathology to confirm the diagnosis, and it is unequivocally a papillary cancer. My recommendation is a total thyroidectomy."

"Tom had the same recommendation, and we are prepared for that surgery. When can you do it? What does your schedule look like?"

"Well, I can do it next Tuesday, I had a cancellation, and we can do it first case. Lauren, you will need to get some pre-op blood work, a chest x-ray, and an EKG. You will also need to see anesthesia. The operation is done under general anesthesia; you will need to be intubated with a breathing tube. The operation takes about two hours. I'll make an elliptical incision across the lower part of your neck. When it heals, you will hardly notice the scar. It is an ambulatory procedure so after you spend a few hours in recovery you will be able to go home. You should not have much pain post-op. Now I need to tell you about one potential problem. Barbara checked your insurance and your policy does not cover the full cost of the operation, and it has no benefit for the anesthesiologist or hospital costs. Were you aware of this?"

"No, you're kidding!"

"Unfortunately, I am not."

I was speechless, although, quite frankly, not surprised.

Lauren worked at BlackRock, one of the largest financial services managers in the world. She had a great job, and was well compensated, but the company gave their employees many options with respect to health insurance coverage. Lauren, like many millennials chose an inexpensive policy reasoning that she was young, healthy, and invincible. Illness, especially a serious illness, is very unlikely in the young adult age group so they throw the dice, take a risk, bet on health, pay lower premiums, and in return increase the amount of take-home dollars in their paychecks. But they set themselves up to get screwed financially if cancer knocks on their door, and they have no option but to let it in. Lauren was screwed, or perhaps better stated, *I* was in serious trouble.

"Hal, give us some time to figure this out and make a few phone calls. Don't give up the OR time next Tuesday, let's see what we can do to figure this out."

"All right, keep me posted, and let me know as soon as you have some information. I will do whatever I can to make the cost palatable as a courtesy, but my hands are tied."

"Understood."

Lauren and I left the office, stunned like deer in the headlights. Now, in addition to having to deal with the cancer, we had the added burden of potentially devastating financial consequences. Healthcare is expensive in the United States, and I really did not want to force my daughter into a clinic environment instead of with doctors and a hospital we knew and trusted.

"When you get to your office, go directly to HR and have a discussion with them; be honest and tell them what you are dealing with and the predicament you face. Ask them to review your policy and see what is possible. I think you should also have a frank discussion with your manager and tell him your diagnosis, that you will need surgery, tests, scans, and that you will miss work for a yet-to-be-determined amount of time. Please tell him everything and mention the insurance issue, and ask if there is anything that can be done."

I honestly believed Lauren would work out this problem with a favorable outcome. She could be relentless with a single-minded focus and would not rest until she achieved her goal. I knew she would be honest and sincere. BlackRock was a tremendous company and extremely supportive of their employees, thus there would be no reason why they would not work with her to change her medical coverage if at all possible, from her current United Health Care Health Maintenance Organization (HMO) to a Preferred Provider Organization (PPO). The former is restrictive, inexpensive, and forces the insured into rigid predetermined doctors and services. The PPO model permits the participant to make choices about doctors, hospitals, and services and, although more expensive, is ultimately the superior coverage.

Lauren called me mid-afternoon. "Dad, Herb called me personally to tell me that all is good. He told me to call the head of HR, and they would make the change for me. They have already started to process the paperwork, and everything should be completed by the end of the week. United will issue me a new insurance card with new member numbers. We need to let Dr. Short know. Will you call him?"

"No, honey you call his office and be certain to make sure that he is planning to do the operation next Tuesday. Do you want to come home to Tenafly tonight?"

"No, I think I am going to go my apartment. I'll be okay. I am also going to go to work for the rest of the week. Our group is working on a big deal and I want to be part of the team. I'll call you and Mom later."

Lauren has come a long way. She is strong; she is ready.

Cancer Machine

Lauren spent the weekend before surgery in her apartment on Central Park South, an iconic street that defines the southern border of Central Park between Fifth Avenue and Columbus Circle. Her building, 265 Central Park South, was adjacent to the Hampshire House Hotel, memorable because my parents, Lucille and Bill, were married there during the final months of World War II; perhaps, more accurately, they were officially married at City Hall by a justice of the peace and had a small family dinner reception at the hotel. Nonetheless, in our family lore, it is a memorable place. The vista above street level, whether winter, spring, summer, or fall, from the buildings that line Central Park South, are breathtakingly beautiful. The Park, framed by Fifth Avenue and Central Park West on the east and west, respectively, spans almost 1,000 acres extending from 59th to 110th Street. The view from Lauren's studio apartment, however, was of internal courtyards and high-rise buildings.

Alicia spoke with Lauren on Saturday afternoon. She was fine, calm, shopping on Madison Avenue with her cousin, Rose Klein, my sister Margaret's middle child. The two girls, three months apart in age, were good friends; they enjoyed the day and were going to have an early dinner at the Candle Café, a vegetarian restaurant. Lauren came home to Tenafly Sunday afternoon and decided not to go to work Monday, but rather spend the day with Alicia to psychologically prepare for surgery. We had dinner at Baumgartens in Englewood, Lauren's choice, the original soda fountain converted Chinese restaurant. We all had our favorite dishes—fried tofu and vegetables for Lauren, shrimp and shallot chips for Alicia, and Kung

Pao chicken for me; homemade ice cream all around for dessert. At dinner, I asked my daughter how she felt and if she had any thoughts.

She replied, "Dad, what choice do I have? I need the surgery."

Her answer resonated with me. I'd heard the exact reply from Herbert Griffo many years ago. Herbert—a tall, blond, handsome, 16-year-old from Staten Island with a wonderful smile and sense of humor—had an osteosarcoma, a malignant bone tumor in his left femur. The night before his scheduled limb-sparing operation, a tumor resection and titanium prosthesis insertion, I asked him if he was prepared for his surgical ordeal, and if he was frightened.

"Doc, what choice do I have?"

I asked him the same question 18 months later when he needed a bilateral thoracotomy to resect multiple metastatic lesions from his lungs.

"Hey, Doc, I trust you. What choice do I have?"

I remember Herbert fondly and spoke with him regularly. He astonishingly survived his cancer and worked on Wall Street as a trader, but became addicted to the narcotics he used to manage his persistent, unrelenting pain and tragically died of a drug overdose. It was heartbreaking after all he had endured.

Honestly, what choice does any cancer patient have? What choice does any patient have when facing a major operation, whether open-heart surgery, gall bladder removal, or a hip replacement? My experience informs that the trepidation is not necessarily due to the operation but the anesthesia; to endure a medically induced sleep and amnesia with total loss of control, one must have total trust in the anesthesiologist. Most surgeries are performed to make patients better, to fix a dysfunctional organ or body part, to relieve pain, to remove an unwanted growth, malignant or benign. What choice do patients really have?

Tuesday morning, we were up early—5 a.m. Lauren was first case and was expected to check-in at 6:30. We showered and dressed; no time for breakfast. I fed and walked Penelope, the family Cavalier King Charles Spaniel. Tension and anxiety were high, conversation forced, no discussion necessary; we were all deep in our solitary thoughts. Lauren acknowledged that she was terrified, but as expected, her fear was the loss of control secondary to the anesthesia.

"Dad, what choice do I have? What if I don't wake up?"

The ride to the hospital from Tenafly was a short 20 minutes. No early morning traffic to contend with. As we traversed the George Washington Bridge, the sun began to rise in the eastern sky, bathing the city in a warm, calming glow. I dropped Lauren and Alicia off in the driveway of the Milstein Hospital building and parked my Audi A6 in the physician's lot on 165th Street. I joined them in the empty lobby. We stopped briefly at the large reception desk, where I presented my Columbia University Medical Center ID and told the security guard that we were expected for surgery check-in. He directed us to the elevators, and we ascended to the third floor and followed the sign to the pre-op reception desk.

Lauren was trembling—her countenance revealed trepidation and panic, yet she walked to the desk, handed her insurance card to the receptionist, completed and signed the necessary documents; the advanced directive, however, regarding instructions should a medical catastrophe occur, alarmed and shocked her. She refused to contemplate the thought and declined to sign the form—her prerogative. The greeter placed an identification band on her left wrist and instructed Lauren to follow signs to the green door, walk through the door to the pre-op intake area where a nurse will explain next steps. She indicated that Alicia and I could join our daughter, so we did.

The intake unit was a large, busy room filled with nurses, nurses' aides, anesthesiologists and surgeons, medical students, residents, and attendings. Everyone had one focus: get the patients checked in and ready to go to the ORs on time with no delays. Mounted from the ceiling were numbers,

1–30. Each signified a patient bay that contained a stretcher for the patient and a straight-back chair for their escort.

"You must be Dr. Weiner, and this is Lauren, yes? I'm Katherine. I'll be your nurse this morning. Go to station 15, I'll be with you in a moment."

Katherine was a large, affable black woman. Intake RNs, by definition, need to be friendly. Their patients, all terrified about what lies ahead, need a strong, compassionate voice for guidance and answers. Katherine handed Lauren two hospital gowns. "Put them both on, the first open to the front and the second open to the back; keep your panties on. Put your clothes in this bag, and let Mom hold your valuables. You can put these cloth slippers on your feet and the head cover over your hair." She handed Lauren what looked like a large white plastic shopping bag with 'New York Presbyterian' emblazoned on it in red letters.

As Katherine took Lauren's vital signs—heart rate, blood pressure, temperature, respiratory rate, and oxygen saturation—Rob Roberts appeared, dressed in green scrubs. Rob and I have been friends at least 40 years. After his pediatric residency, he completed a second residency in anesthesiology at Columbia and remained on staff as a faculty member. Roberts primarily worked with the urologists, providing service to patients requiring prostate, bladder, and kidney surgery. Nevertheless, I asked him to provide anesthesia to Lauren for her thyroidectomy. I trusted him—he was careful, conservative, and experienced, and I figured his engaging, outgoing personality would help her relax, if possible.

Rob introduced himself to Lauren in a calm, measured voice, explaining every detail from beginning to end. Rob told her that he would escort her from the pre-op area into the operating room theater. He told her that he would insert an IV into her arm to facilitate delivery of medication. He told her he would monitor her heart and respiratory function throughout the entire operation. He told her he would put her to sleep by administering Propofol and Ketamine intravenously. He told her she would need to be intubated with a breathing tube inserted into her trachea, but she would be asleep. He told her he would not leave her side during the surgery and when she awoke, he would be the first person she would see.

Rob asked, "Has Dr. Short been here yet?"

As if summoned, Hal appeared, dressed in a gray suit, white shirt, and red Hermès tie decorated with racehorses. "Good morning, Weiner family." He extended his hand to Lauren and spoke directly to her. He reviewed his intent to perform a total thyroidectomy and demonstrated on her neck where he would make the incision. He explained the risk of inadvertently removing one of the four parathyroid glands and the complication of tetany should this occur. He told Lauren that the entire operation would take less than two hours, and after a few hours rest in the recovery room she would be able to go home. Hal handed Lauren the consent form for the surgery, and she signed it without hesitation.

Dad, what choice do I have?

Hal said, "Lauren, I'll see you in the OR. I have to change."

Dr. Roberts asked Lauren if she was ready. "Let's go. Michael, I have your mobile number, so I'll call you as soon as we're done."

Alicia and I gave our little girl a kiss and, escorted by Rob Roberts, she disappeared through the door into the belly of the operating rooms. It was a surreal, out-of-body experience. Despite the knowledge that Lauren was in superb hands with the best doctors, I was unable to prevent the thought that, although rare, accidental mishaps occur during even the most innocuous surgeries, and patients die.

I recall describing to Anne Oliver, Bill's mother, my thoughts about Lauren and watching her disappear into the world of operating rooms, anesthesia machines, overhead lights, sterile tables, and patients completely covered by sterile gowns except for the surgical field. Anne was similarly terrified, as every parent would be, as she watched her son disappear into the OR the morning Jordan Klein performed a thoracotomy to remove the NUT midline carcinoma. I tried to convince Anne that her reaction and emotion were quite an appropriate reaction for any parent. Alicia and I clearly did.

As Dr. Roberts expertly administered anesthesia to allow Dr. Short to deftly remove her cancerous thyroid gland, Alicia and I went to the Milstein cafeteria on the second floor for a bagel and coffee. We then went to my office on Irving-7 to relax for a few minutes. I read a few emails. It was early—7:30 in the morning—so the floor was empty. At 8:15, we walked to the surgery designated visitor lounge, a large, windowless room with uncomfortable neutral colored chairs on the third floor of Milstein just off the elevator lobby. We each took a section of *The New York Times* and feigned reading.

My mobile phone vibrated at 8:50. Rob Roberts said, "We're all done. Short was masterful. Lauren will be in recovery in 15 minutes. I'll look for you there; it's on the fourth floor."

"Thanks, Rob."

Lauren looked great, if a bit pale, with a small bandage on her neck. She was certainly comfortable at the moment. Dr. Short approached Lauren's bed; smiling, he told us that the operation went extremely well. There had been no issues, no concerns. He indicated that he removed one sub-centimeter lymph node that went to surgical pathology with intact resected thyroid gland. Hal told Lauren that she could shower in two to three days, gave her a prescription for Toradol, should she have pain, and Synthroid, thyroid hormone replacement, 125 micrograms daily. He told Lauren to call the office and make an appointment to see him in 10 days.

We were home by early afternoon. Lauren slept in the guest room with Penelope curled at the foot of the bed, guarding her from intruders. She experienced little pain, and recovery was relatively easy and uneventful.

Short called to tell Lauren that the pathology confirmed papillary thyroid carcinoma and that the removed lymph node was positive for cancer. Interestingly, we learned there was no prognostic significance to the positive lymph node; this finding is the only cancer where this phenomenon exists. In every other disease, a positive lymph node indicates metastatic spread and mandates more intensive treatment.

Tom James called to inquire how Lauren was recuperating and told her to stop by after her appointment with Short. He explained the need for a total body thyroid scan with radioactive iodine (RAI) to determine if any aberrant thyroid tissue existed. The test was a simple injection and scan; however, the preparation for the test was onerous, two weeks of an iron-free diet; very restrictive and tasteless—no meat, fish, legumes, non-iodized salt . . . the list of food to be omitted is long.

We learned that there is another approach: Thyrogen (thyrotropin alfa) is a protein identical to natural human thyroid-stimulating hormone (TSH), a hormone produced by the pituitary gland in your brain that tells your thyroid to make and release thyroid hormones into the bloodstream. Thyrogen is given in two injections prior to radioactive iodine ablation or diagnostic testing in patients with well-differentiated papillary thyroid cancer. Thyrogen raises the levels of TSH in your body, which is important when preparing for RAI ablation or a diagnostic scan.

Columbia does not have Thyrogen readily available, which is hard to believe considering it is one of the great academic medical centers in the world. With James' consent, we made an appointment to see Mark Tyson at Sloan Kettering.

Memorial Sloan Kettering is an enigma to me. I'm not certain why; it just is. I have had several opportunities at multiple junctures in my career to work at MSK and, for some reason, always chose another path. Something about the place—arrogance, dominance, bravado—did not resonate with me. But Dr. Tyson was widely respected and offered Thyrogen, thus, as a family, we went for Lauren.

Located on York Avenue and 68th Street, directly across the avenue from New York Presbyterian Weill Cornell, MSK presents an imposing image. It is crowded with cancer patients, in the lobby, on the escalator, in the cafeteria, crowding onto elevators, people everywhere. The patients were identifiable; they were hairless or wore hats and scarfs to cover their bald heads. Tyson's office was on the eighth floor of the ambulatory building. The shared waiting room was large with stark, windowless walls devoid of color and uncomfortable chairs lacking humanity.

A nurse called Lauren's name and escorted us into Tyson's office. He was pleasant, welcoming. He was up-to-date on her history, having previously reviewed the medial record, op report, and pathology from Columbia. He confirmed the need for the RAI scan and discussed the need for thyroid ablation using a radioactive isotope. He indicated two approaches, low dose ablation versus high dose, explaining the merits of each. Low-dose has less toxicity but increased risk of recurrence, perhaps approaching 30 percent. High-dose RAI has heightened risk of infertility, second cancers, lethargy, pulmonary fibrosis and xerostomia, and dry mouth, but a markedly decreased risk of relapse—well less than five percent.

Cancer is never cut and dried. There are always decisions to be made, questions to answer, risk, reward. There is never ever an obvious path forward without repercussion.

Lauren and I immersed ourselves in amateur Google research, as we had previously, to learn as much about radioactive iodine treatment as possible. We resorted to lay information—her charge and medical literature, my responsibility. We learned that although the side effects were real, not imagined, the probability of infertility and second malignancies was quite low, in the range of one to two cases out of a hundred. Considering the alternative—a significantly greater relapse rate—the decision was apparent.

"Dad, I want the high-dose treatment."

After reviewing the facts, I agreed completely. The most terrifying words a cancer patient or parent of a patient must endure: "Your cancer has recurred!"

The diagnostic scan was now complete and resulted without evidence of aberrant thyroid tissue. Dr. Tyson scheduled the RAI ablation for a Monday morning.

Lauren was cool and very matter-of-fact. "Let's get this done. I'm gonna beat this cancer."

Shockingly, I heard that precise protestation before. My father, William, enjoyed excellent health until the age of 92, at which time he experienced life-altering, threatening illnesses—diffuse large B-cell non-Hodgkin's lymphoma and a renal cell carcinoma. He received eight months of chemotherapy for the lymphoma and a nephrectomy for the latter. He survived both malignancies. At the age of 95, he fell, hit his head, developed a subdural hematoma in his brain, had a seizure, and required emergency surgery at JFK Hospital in Atlantis, Florida. The post-op care at JFK was abysmal—about the worst I have witnessed. There was no doctor managing his care, only a nurse. We were able to have an air ambulance, at great expense, fly him to Teterboro, New Jersey, and then transport him to the neuro ICU at Columbia. The care there was superb, and he survived. One morning, grabbing my hand, my father said out of the corner of his contorted mouth, "I'm gonna beat this." He survived and lived another 18 months.

Now my daughter professed the identical statement of desire, strength, fortitude, and will to live: "I'm gonna beat this."

The RAI ablation is performed in Nuclear Medicine. After registration and signing the obligatory documents and consents, Dr. Osaki explained the procedure. Lauren would receive 120 microcuries of radioactive iodine, a simple injection, followed by a scan. The entire treatment would take about two and a half hours. Afterwards, Lauren could go home but would have to be in a room alone for a minimum of 72 hours. She would be slightly radioactive and emit gamma rays that are potentially harmful to others. She could have no contact with family members or pets, taking meals in the room. Osaki told her that she could use the bathroom but should be the only person to have access to the commode for the three-day period as the radiation is found in urine and stool.

As Lauren received her treatment, Alicia and I walked to Bloomingdale's on Third Avenue. We bought nothing; we were just killing time. We stopped for lunch at a small neighborhood bistro. Upon returning to Nuclear Medicine to retrieve our daughter, the technician told us to get our car and pull in front of the main entrance on York Avenue and a transporter would bring Lauren downstairs to meet us.

Our daughter looked great, felt great, and was thrilled to have the ordeal behind her. She rigidly followed the doctor's orders, staying in total isolation for 72 hours without Penelope. She stayed in Tenafly about a week and then returned to her apartment and to work at BlackRock.

After all, what choice did she have?

She won. Her thyroid cancer was defeated. She "beat this."

Follow-up was relatively routine and innocuous—regular visits to Tom James for exams, neck sonograms, and blood work to monitor her TSH level. The desired number is 0–1, total suppression of thyroid function by the exogenous daily Synthroid; Lauren has continuously been in this range.

One afternoon, several years after her diagnosis of thyroid cancer, Lauren called my cell crying. "Dad, I'm a cancer machine."

At a recent routine visit to her gynecologist, Bruce Barry had conducted a Pap smear, a procedure to test for cervical cancer, and it had come back positive. The test involves collecting cells from the cervix, the lower, narrow end of the uterus at the top of the vagina, and examining for cellular atypia and pre-malignant conditions. The test also reports the presence or absence of Human Papilloma Virus, HPV, a common sexually transmitted virus associated with cervical cancer. Lauren was positive for serotypes 16 and 18, variants associated with more than 75 percent chance of cervical cancer.

I was shocked and horrified; concerned not for the positive test—I knew procedures existed to manage this scenario—but the psycho-emotional effect that had the potential to wreak havoc. HPV is ubiquitous, common, and unrelated to thyroid cancer, yet Lauren had to address its presence, and complications were possible.

The following morning at 7 a.m., Bruce Barry and I attended a Columbia Doctors Executive committee meeting in the dean's conference room on the second floor of the Physicians and Surgeons Medical School building. Columbia Doctors is the faculty practice organization and the executive committee, five department chairs and four non-chairs, is charged with setting policy and governing the more than 1,500 physicians who provide patient care. At the conclusion of the meeting, I asked Bruce about Lauren. He told me nothing that I did not already know, explaining the pre-malignant cellular dysplasia and the HPV positivity on the Pap smear.

"Michael, your daughter will be fine—don't worry."

Bruce Barry and his wife, Kayla, were a quintessential New York power couple. Bruce cared for and delivered the babies of many of the city's influential and important women. Kayla, an editorial director of Hearst Magazines and literary consultant, was highly regarded in her field and wielded significant influence. Together they attended important premieres at Lincoln Center, Carnegie Hall, and participated in all the correct charitable foundations; they were A-listers. The Barrys owned an old farmhouse in Wassaic, New York, not far from our home in Salisbury, Connecticut. Bruce, Evan Cole, and I rode our bikes on the rail trail in Millerton. Away from the hospital with his guard down, Bruce was fun, had a dry sense of humor, and in spandex bike shorts, was one of the boys.

Lauren asked me to accompany her the day of her appointment with Dr. Barry for colposcopy and a loop electrosurgical excision, LEEP. The former provides a magnified exam of the cervix, vagina, and vulva for signs of disease. In the latter, a thin wire loop that carries an electric current is used to remove abnormal areas of the cervix. The technique is performed in the office, utilizing local anesthesia with topical lidocaine—a relatively painless 15 minutes.

Bruce was pleased with the procedure and confident that he'd removed involved pre-cancerous lesions. The LEEP has a small risk of gestational problems, however, Dr. Barry having performed the procedure on hundreds of patients, felt assured that the lining of Lauren's cervix was not violated.

Post colposcopy and LEEP, Lauren felt fine physically and, surprisingly, emotionally as well. Rather than spending the night in Tenafly, she chose to take a cab to her apartment. I was relieved.

Lauren was strong, a survivor. She conquered thyroid cancer and similarly prevailed against the threat of cervical cancer. She married, had two uneventful pregnancies, no complications from the radioactive iodine or LEEP, and has a perfect family—a boy and a girl.

Bruce Barry and Evan Cole continued to bike ride, but I stopped. One day on the rail trail while crossing a road, I was hit by a car and broke four ribs. No more biking for me. I bought a Peloton instead.

Several years later, I received a terrifying phone call from Evan. "Bruce Barry is dead."

They were riding together, Bruce swerved to avoid hitting a walker on the trail, tumbled over the handlebar, hit his head, and fractured his pelvis. When the ambulance arrived, he was seizing, had a massive intracranial hemorrhage, went into cardiac arrest, and could not be resuscitated.

Kayla, unfortunately, did not appreciate that Bruce was gone. She had developed severe dementia and did not remember her husband and partner of 50 years. Honestly, she did not even know her own name.

Life is cruel, unfair.

Baruch Hashem

We arrived in the Central Pediatric Intensive Care Unit out of breath, having run up the back stairs rather than waiting for the elevator. We had sensed that something was wrong with Harris Schulman. Although always frenetic, the world of beeps, flashing lights, medical technology, and machines felt particularly abrasive in this moment. There was already a group of people congregated outside of Room 912, Harris' room. His oxygen saturation had dropped to a dangerously low level, which had caused his heart rate to slow precipitously. Nurses and doctors were at the bedside administering medications and adjusting the respirator settings in order to stabilize his condition. Dr. Roger Carroll, the Director of the Division of Pediatric Critical Care, was directing his disciples and leading the process. Each member of the team had a specific role.

Patient rounds in the PICU are interesting. The team is large; at times it reaches 7 to 10 people. Harris' bedside nurse, Carol Vasquez, reported his vital signs, respirator settings, oxygen saturation, and urine output—all important data needed for decision-making. Arthur Smith, the critical care clinical fellow, and Debbie Haverford, a second-year resident, reviewed the medication list, recent laboratory data, and viewed the recent chest x-ray on the mobile computer screen. Listening, observing, and learning, were two third-year medical students and the on-call critical care physician assistant, Valerie Schocat. I was present and available to provide insight to the group should issues arise surrounding leukemia and its specific management, but Carroll was in charge. Mr. Schulman joined the conversation and listened intently. We generally encourage the parents of patients in the

ICU to participate in the conversation and decision-making process and ask as many questions as they need in order to understand the often-complex procedures.

Carroll, acknowledging the presence of the oncology team, indicated that decisions needed to be made. He told us that they were having difficulty providing Harris with sufficient oxygenation despite maximum ventilator settings and 100 percent inspired oxygen. He suggested introducing ECMO and wanted our input.

I turned to Lisa Jones, our leukemia team nurse practitioner, and Charlie, a first-year fellow. "What do you guys think we should do? Should we begin ECMO?"

Charlie was a fellow, specializing in pediatric hematology-oncology. He was raised in Coral Gables, Florida. His parents, both former New Yorkers, met in college at the University of Florida in Gainesville, moved to the Miami area after graduation, and never left. His dad was an attorney and his mother was an early preschool educator. Charlie graduated from MIT where he also played basketball. Who would have guessed that the top-ranked engineering and technology school in the country even had a basketball team? Apparently they do, and Charlie started at guard. He went to medical school in Israel and completed his residency at the Nicklaus Children's Hospital in Miami.

I remember interviewing Charlie when he applied for fellowship; I liked him immediately. I answered his obligatory questions about call schedules, clinical responsibilities, and research opportunities, but mostly we talked about basketball. We had both been undersized point guards on small, Division III basketball teams and were in complete agreement about how woefully terrible the New York Knicks were, season after season. We spoke the same language.

Our team desperately needed a male in the program; all of our fellows at the time were women. Within the last decade, pediatrics and pediatric hematology-oncology has become a female-dominated sub-specialty, a positive evolution, as female physicians generally possess outstanding compassion, knowledge, and leadership capabilities. On the other hand, Charlie did not disappoint. He was hard-working, cared deeply about his patients, had good judgment, and was eager to learn. During the third year of his fellowship he was appointed Chief Fellow, assumed and exceeded all expectations administratively, and emerged as a bona fide clinical investigator.

"Yes," he said. "We should begin ECMO."

"Why?"

"He has a curable underlying disease, acute lymphoblastic leukemia, ALL. Pneumocystis jirovecii is also potentially curable if we can support him and allow the antibiotics to work."

"I agree," I said. "Let's do it. Roger, we are putting Harris' care in your capable hands with the expertise of your unit."

Mr. Schulman, Harris' father, was listening to the conversation and asked, "Can you explain to me what pneum . . . pneumo . . . forgive me but I cannot pronounce the word. And what is ECMO?"

Mr. Schulman was a portly man who dressed in the obligatory garb of Hasidic men—black baggy pants, black shoes, white shirt, black vest, and a *yarmulke*. He had lost his wife to breast cancer about a year prior, and now his son had leukemia and was fighting for his life. The family had a very strong cancer history. Harris' mother had four sisters. She and one of her sisters both had breast and uterine cancer and were deceased. The third sister had just been diagnosed with ovarian cancer and was reportedly BRCA mutation positive, meaning that, genetically, she was five times more likely than the average woman to develop breast and ovarian cancer. Mr. Schulman's side of the family had fared no better. Both of his brothers had been diagnosed with pancreatic cancer, and both were deceased.

Mr. Schulman was a very kind, simple man. His devotion to his son was evident; he was at the hospital early each morning and spent the entire day by his side, only leaving in the evening to sleep at his home in Williamsburg before returning to the hospital first thing the next morning. When the Sabbath began on Friday night he remained at his son's bedside until its conclusion on Saturday at sundown. He repeated this routine day after day and week after week for his son's entire 47-day hospital stay. He was a stoic person, showing no emotion. He wanted to know only what he needed to know and was satisfied in his belief that the doctors and nurses were doing all they could to save his son's life. He spent most of the day reading from a little black book of prayers and psalms. His demeanor was consistent with the Hasidic culture—caring yet reserved, and steadfast in the believe that God will protect and heal.

Dr. Ruth Goldstein, the New York Presbyterian Hospital epidemiologist and a pediatric infectious disease expert, joined the discussion. I have known Ruth for 25 years and have always enjoyed working with her. She was tall with short, cropped, dark hair, and the pockets of her white coat were always jam-packed with notes, handbooks, and recent references. I appreciated her quiet and thoughtful manner and trusted her judgment explicitly. She was and is a delight to work with.

Ruth addressed Mr. Schulman: "Pneumocystis is a type of infection that primarily affects patients with a compromised immune system, such as people with HIV/AIDS, or in your son's case, secondary to chemotherapy, in particular, steroids such as dexamethasone. The cause is an unusual type of fungus that primarily affects the lungs. When did you notice that something was wrong? When did Harris become ill?"

"Well, three days ago he started coughing and had a fever. I brought him to the emergency room Sunday morning after *Shabbos* and he was having difficulty breathing. They did a chest x-ray and admitted him immediately to the intensive care unit."

"Was he taking his Bactrim?"

Bactrim is an antibiotic that is used not only to treat pneumocystis, but also is used prophylactically to prevent infection.

"Harris is almost 20 years old, he is responsible, takes his own medicine, and said he did not miss any dosages. I believe and trust him. So, as far as I can tell, he was taking it. Why do you ask?"

Ruth Goldstein explained that Bactrim prophylaxis taken twice a day for three days a week has been shown to prevent a serious pneumocystis infection. In fact, since cancer patients began taking Bactrim, the incidence of the infection has been significantly reduced.

Dr. Carroll intervened. "Right now, Harris is really sick. He has a severe lung infection, is respirator-dependent, has liver and kidney failure, and there is tremendous pressure on his heart to pump blood to his organs and brain."

"Dr. Weiner, is my son going to die?" Mr. Schulman turned to me, his damp eyes betraying the emotion beneath his stoic façade. "Promise me you will not allow this to happen."

I was Harris' primary oncologist. I had performed the original bone marrow aspirate, biopsy, and lumbar puncture to confirm the diagnosis, obtained consent for therapy, guided the treatment, and was present at all of his outpatient visits. Harris and his dad trusted me. It was my responsibility to tell Mr. Schulman that his son was critically ill. I emphasized that Harris would receive the best care available from the doctors and nurses in the intensive care unit.

I told Mr. Schulman that Dr. Carroll's team was unequivocally among the very best in the country, had access to the most modern technology, and would do everything necessary to bring his son back from the euphemistic "jaws of death." Most significantly, I told him that Harris' leukemia was in remission and that his present precarious state was secondary to pneumocystis jirovecii, an overwhelming yeast-like fungal infection. We expected him to survive, but knew that it would take time, patience, state of the art medical management, and high dosages of the specific antibiotic, Bactrim.

"Patients similar to Harris *do* make it. You have my word that with God's help he will make it."

Mr. Schulman took my hand. "*Baruch Hashem*. Thank you."

Thirty or so years ago, while I was working at Mt. Sinai Hospital, I recall caring for a very ill, young Hasidic girl. I told her parents that I believed that their daughter would not live through the night. Her mother became enraged with me, telling me that doctors do not make decisions about life and death, only God makes such decisions, *not you—how dare you!*

I was embarrassed and mortified. I never before realized or appreciated how deep faith in God influenced every thought, every action, every decision; the omnipotent nature of the Almighty was foreign to me—it was not in my DNA. I do believe in God and often silently pray for assistance and guidance, but the extreme devotion and paralysis of the Hasidic sect is beyond my comprehension. I accept it, but do not understand it.

That conversation shaped the way that I speak to Hasidic families. They are deeply religious, pray constantly, and believe that God's will is supreme and is not to be questioned. They view doctors as messengers of God, vehicles of the Almighty who are sent to do his work with the sick.

The Hasidic movement was founded by Rabbi Israel Baal Shem Tov in the early 1700s in what is today the Ukraine. Its original teachings were of peace, joy, humility, and charity. A Hasid, then, is one who strives to become a better person and a better servant of God, through study of the Bible and the Talmud, which is the central text of Rabbinic Judaism and is the primary source of Jewish religious law and theology. There exist many different Hasidic sects in the United States, primarily located in and around the New York metropolitan area. Additional Hasidic concentrations exist in the east coast cities of Boston, Philadelphia, and Miami, as well as Chicago and Los Angeles. In New York, the group is further subdivided into branches in Borough Park, Crown Heights, and Williamsburg in Brooklyn and Monsey, and Monroe in Rockland County, north of the city. The Schulman family is from Williamsburg.

Unflappable is the word I would use to describe Dr. Roger Carroll. I suspect that caring exclusively for critically ill patients with acute and chronic life-threatening diseases has a way of stabilizing one's constitution. His ability to present a calm demeanor to patients and families, not to mention his trainees, is a tremendous professional asset. Perhaps his character evolved from his early years in Washington state, surrounded by the kind of overwhelming natural grandeur that necessarily instills perspective, a sense of one's scale in the world, and the frivolity of so much of what we as humans stress over. He also completed his education on the west coast, including medical school at Stanford, which although superb and competitive, has a more relaxed vibe than the New York and other east coast schools. Roger had inherited the sort of calm assuredness that can't be taught. It's something that many doctors aspire to and all patients are drawn to, whether they are able to name it or not.

At the completion of Roger's training, he joined the faculty at the University of Texas Southwestern in Dallas. I was a member of a search committee charged with hiring a new director of our division of critical care, and Roger Carroll was, without question, the single best candidate we considered. Columbia and our Department of Pediatrics were, and are, lucky to have him on our faculty. He and his wife Beth moved to Larchmont, a Westchester County suburb, under an hour north of the city. Their son, John, has Down's syndrome, and although relatively well, has had medical issues, and I am certain that this experience has also helped shape Roger's approach to patients and families.

During rounds, Dr. Carroll was in total control of both his team and the management of the patients. He was casually dressed in an open-collar blue shirt and beige chinos. He sat at the computer screen mounted on a movable stand, reviewing all the labs, and listening to the nurses and residents present an update of the previous night's events and Harris' status. He was entirely focused on the numbers: heart rate, blood pressure, respiratory rate, intake and output of fluids, oxygen and carbon dioxide levels, and the lab results for blood counts, electrolytes, liver function, and renal function tests. In critically ill patients, the numbers tell the story.

I walked into Harris' room, struggling to comprehend the state of my patient. There was a smell of blood, sterile air, alcohol, and fear. Laying in his hospital bed, Harris Schulman was motionless; medically paralyzed to maximize the effects of the respirator. Tape secured the breathing tube in his throat and kept his eyes shut to prevent drying of his corneas. His thin, frail body belied the fact that just two weeks ago he had been extremely well; his leukemia had been responding to treatment, his blood counts were normal, and he was on the path to cure. He had been a robust 18-year-old—quiet, reserved, trusting, and barely communicative as most Hasidic teenagers are, but pleasant, and evidently healthy.

This morning, however, Harris' numbers had shown a deteriorating trend—concrete evidence of multiple organ failure. His lungs, liver, and kidneys were weakening and could no longer sustain life. We were losing our battle. We needed a heroic measure. We needed ECMO, extracorporeal membrane oxygenation, a mechanical technique of providing prolonged cardiac and respiratory support to persons whose heart and lungs are unable to provide an adequate amount of oxygen and carbon dioxide exchange or perfusion to support life. It is used to counter late-stage situations of severe heart and lung failure, when recovery is deemed possible and the underlying condition treatable.

Dr. Carroll told Mr. Schulman, "By utilizing the ECMO now, we will be better able to support Harris. It will allow time for the antibiotics to eradicate the lung infection, and allow the respirator to better breathe for him, reducing the very significant stress on his heart and lungs; he needs a rest, and we have the technology to allow this to happen. We need to call the surgeons to place a canula in his femoral artery and call the respiratory therapy team to connect Harris to the machine. We need you to sign a consent in order for us to proceed."

"I need to make a few phone calls," Mr. Schulman replied, betraying no emotion. "I need a few minutes to think. Dr. Weiner, do you agree with this drastic approach?"

"Yes, I do. It is the correct decision. Do you want me to speak to Gitti Goldberg and the Rebbe to inform and solicit their approval?"

Mr. Schulman and Harris trusted me. I believe this had less to do with the fact that I was Jewish and more to do with my proven record of care for Harris and my commitment to keeping Mr. Schulman as well informed and comfortable as possible, given the circumstances. Still, my being Jewish couldn't have hurt. I often give patients my cell phone number and instruct them to call me if they have questions or issues, regardless of how insignificant they may seem. I would prefer to deal with problems as they arise, in the moment, rather than allow such matters to fester. I have found patients and families to be respectful—they call infrequently—but the offer alone helps to solidify our relationship. This is of paramount importance when treating children and adolescents with grave illnesses. Patients deserve physicians who are fully and completely involved in every aspect of their care.

"Yes," Mr. Schulman said. "Let's call Gitti Goldberg and the Rebbe."

We walked to a small conference room just off the elevator lobby on the ninth floor. I knew that Mrs. Goldberg and the Rebbe would agree with our suggested course of action. Culturally, the ultra-Orthodox discuss all important decisions with their advisors and community elders, but in cases like this, it was really a formality, though a necessary one. Schulman dialed the emergency phone number of Refuah Helpline, whose primary function is to provide aid to Orthodox Jewish and Hasidic people seeking medical advice, referrals, and assistance in making expedited appointments with healthcare providers. His call was answered by an answering service, so he left a message.

"Let me call Gitti Goldberg on her cell phone," I said. "I am certain she won't mind. We speak at all hours of the day and night." I dialed the number, and she answered on the first ring. "Gitti, how are you?"

"*Baruch Hashem*, thank God," she answered.

"I am sitting with Mr. Schulman, Harris' father, and we want to ask your advice. Harris is critically ill, and Dr.Carroll, the Director of the PICU, wants to put him on ECMO. We wanted to let you know and also to get your approval."

"Of course. I agree. Whatever Dr.Carroll thinks is best."

"Thank you, Gitti. Be well."

Gitti Goldberg leads the Refuah Helpline. Her Rolodex has the names, office contacts, and cell phone numbers of hundreds of doctors, primarily across New York City. For a physician, membership in the Refuah Helpline referral list is a big deal. It's a badge of honor and a sign of excellence.

I visited the Refuah office in Monroe, New York with my esteemed colleagues, Daniel Hito and Constantine Drakos, on an unseasonably warm October afternoon. Mrs. Goldberg and her minions were in a festive mood, having recently celebrated Rosh Hashanah and Yom Kippur, the Jewish New Year and Day of Atonement, respectively, and Sukkot, a festival of the harvest.

The community is an isolated enclave of extreme orthodoxy located 30 miles northwest of the city, not far from Woodbury Commons, one of the largest discount outlet shopping malls in the country. Every building and every house in this modern-day ghetto look nearly identical: beige, four-story wood structures with white shutters. There were hundreds of these houses, each edifice home to a single extended family of two to three generations. It is quite common for a family to have 10 to 12 children; each one considered a blessing from God. Thus, grandparents who are often in their mid to late forties might have 100 or more grandchildren.

The day we visited the temperature was near 70 degrees. School children were everywhere, and one could not help but observe that the boys, dressed in black and white with skull caps on their heads, stayed separate from the girls, who all wore long plaid skirts and white blouses, and had ribbons in their hair. The girls' youth contrasted their garb, evocative of a time long past.

From childhood, contact between male and female members of the Hasidic sects is strictly forbidden. At school, they are in separate classrooms, and at *shul*, or synagogue, the center of community life, they are separated as well; the men are downstairs and the women, girls, and boys younger than 13 years of age (before Bar Mitzvah) are upstairs. Needless to say, while women like Gitti Goldberg have managed to forge leadership roles within the community, modern feminism is not a pillar of Hasidic Judaism.

Street after street in Monroe were identical in appearance, the street signs written in Yiddish, the language spoken by the Hasidim. The signs on the ShopRite Supermarket and the CVS were in both Yiddish and English. If you closed your eyes and applied a bit of imagination, you could almost envision the ghettos of pre-World War II Warsaw or Prague.

Hanna's office was a structure like the others. On the small patch of grass in the front courtyard sat a large sign, written, of course, in both Yiddish and English, which read "REFUAH HELPLINE." This was not, strictly speaking, an office building, but Gitti's home, with the central operating hub located on the first floor alongside a foyer, kitchen, dining room, living room, and several smaller rooms that were retrofit to accommodate personnel. The living room was a large space, divided into cubicles, each with a chair, desk, computer screen, and phone. The room was a beehive of activity; behind each desk, a female volunteer.

Gitti, dressed modestly in a very simple long skirt covering her legs, a clashing colorful blouse, and a tight-fitting head covering, greeted us with her assistant, Hashe, in tow. Hashe wore traditional Hasidic garb: a long black coat with a white shirt and a wide-brimmed black hat.

Though I've known Gitti for about 15 years, I honestly do not know what possessed her to become a medical referral liaison for her community; perhaps she had a child or family member that was ill and struggled to find appropriate care for them. But regardless of her motivation, she serves a vital function for her community. I am 100 percent certain that she has no formal medical training whatsoever—not even as an allied health provider. Her knowledge is superficial, but she knows a little about a lot of conditions. More important for the community is her little black book, her long list of physicians who will respond to her outreach at any time, day or night. Thus, if she hears that a particular patient has heart disease, breast cancer, childhood leukemia, or needs a spine surgeon, she knows who to call.

Gitti and Hashe escorted us into the dining room, where a table was lavishly set for lunch with fine china, cloth napkins, sterling silver cutlery, and a center piece of plastic faux flowers. Daniel, Constantine, and I took our seats with the community religious dignitaries, Refuah Helpline leadership, and Drs. Wasserman, a father and son team who provided pediatric care to the community.

The men sat at the main table, and Gitti and three other women sat separated from the men at a folding bridge table to the side. Lunch was a feast of six courses, including matzah ball soup, stuffed derma (a delicacy made from beef intestine casing stuffed with vegetables), salad, roast chicken with potatoes, and dessert. I ate virtually nothing. The luncheon meal, though abundant, was remarkably tasteless. Daniel and Constantine also politely pushed the offering from one side of the plate to the other. We picked.

The conversation was courteous, and we re-enforced our desire to care for Hasidic children with cancer at Columbia. We promised to be respectful, prompt, and communicative, and to provide attentive management, regardless of the patient and family's ability to pay.

Roger Carroll joined us. "We need to move quickly," he said. "The surgeons are at Harris' bedside and ready to insert the cannulas into the femoral artery in his groin. We need you to sign the consent form now."

"I have no choice, do I?"

"You do not."

Staring blankly, with no expression of emotion, Mr. Schulman reached into his pocket for a pen and signed the consent. "Dr. Weiner, I still want to call the Rebbe and at least inform him of what we are doing."

"Absolutely, who is your Rebbe?"

In the Hasidic tradition a Rebbe, or Rabbi, is the leader of the sect. Each sect, or group, has their own unique individual who provides spiritual guidance, mentorship, and consultations regarding every aspect of life, from the mundane to the life changing. The followers of a Rebbe ask for his approval whenever a major decision confronts them. Whether or not to place Harris on ECMO rises to the level of requiring permission; it is a decision that involves life and death. As a leader of his flock, the Rebbe commands similar devotion and reverence as the Pope and Dalai Lama do for their followers.

Mr. Schulman dialed the phone number of Rabbi Ausch, his Rebbe in Williamsburg. "This is Mr. Schulman, father of Harris. May I speak to the Rabbi?"

"Rabbi Ausch is not available. What is your call about?"

"My son is very sick at the intensive care unit at Columbia Medical Center, and I must inform the Rabbi of his condition and ask his permission for the doctors to do a special procedure."

"Mr. Schulman, give me your cell number, and I will have the Rabbi get right back to you."

"*Baruch Hashem.*" With God's help.

Mr. Schulman's cell phone rang within minutes.

"This is Rabbi Ausch."

"Rabbi, I am sitting with Dr. Weiner, Harris' doctor, I am going to put you on speakerphone so he can join the conversation."

"Hello Rabbi," I said. "How are you?"

"*Baruch Hashem.*"

"Rabbi, Harris Schulman is desperately ill, and we need to put him on ECMO, a type of life support. We wanted you to know, and to agree with, the plan."

"Of course," the Rabbi agreed, as I had expected he would. "Keep me posted. We will pray for Harris and for all the doctors and nurses."

We walked back into the PICU. Dr. Carroll and his team had moved to the next room to help a teenage boy who had been in an automobile accident and had multiple trauma. He was post-op and would survive; the jury remained out on Harris Schulman. Bob Jones, a pediatric surgeon, had just finished placing the ECMO cannulas in the left femoral artery and vein, as the nurses and perfusion technician were injecting heparin into the circuit to keep it from clotting. They were ready to turn the system on, and when Bob pressed the power button, a whirring sound indicated that all systems were a go.

I stopped for a moment to take it all in. The ICU room was relatively large as far as hospital rooms go. There was a sink to the left with canisters of hand sanitizer and soap attached to the wall. To the right was a pullout day bed with a dark blue faux mattress for a parent if they wished to stay the night.

Harris lay in the bed in the center of the room. An endotracheal tube was taped in his mouth, attached to the breathing apparatus. Coming out of his nose was a nasogastric tube, through which he could be fed high-caloric liquid nutrients; this too was taped to secure its placement. His eyes were covered with tape to keep them closed to prevent the corneas from becoming dry. He had a Foley catheter in his penis in order to accurately measure his urine output. There was tubing in his right wrist called an arterial line, which allowed measurement of the blood gases needed to assess the respirator settings. There was a large dialysis catheter in his right femoral vein to cleanse his system of toxic blood components because his kidneys were not working effectively. Connected to the PORT, the venous access device in his chest, were intravenous lines to provide antibiotics, medications, and transfusions of red blood cells and platelets. The newly cannulated catheter for the ECMO was placed in his left groin.

As I stood in the doorway looking at my desperately ill patient, I was incredulous. The body in the bed was not human; it had a name, but its humanness, its heart and soul, were elsewhere in the ether. Harris was heavily sedated and paralyzed out of necessity—if he survived, he would not remember the ordeal, which was most assuredly a good thing. Mr. Schulman sat in the corner of the room, reciting prayers and psalms from his black book.

Who Lives? Who Dies?

For patients hospitalized in an intensive care unit, time seems suspended. There is a monotonous rhythm of stagnation, minutes become hours, hours become days, and days become weeks. Such was the situation with Harris Schulman, but this tedious ordeal was necessary for Harris and similar patients in order to reverse the downward spiral and survive. There is a defined progression from stability to slow improvement to wellness. Harris was stable. The interventions initiated by Dr. Carroll seemed to be working, at least for the moment.

I visited Harris and his father often, but my bedside stays were social, more for moral support; we talked about the weather. Mr. Schulman told me he was recently remarried and worked as an EMT for the Brooklyn branch of the local Hatzalah, a volunteer emergency medical service organization serving Jewish communities around the world. My role as his primary oncologist, for the moment, was minimal, almost non-existent.

One day, Mr. Schulman asked, "Is it safe for Harris not to receive his chemotherapy?"

I replied, "Chemotherapy at this time is too dangerous, contraindicated."

I explained to Harris' father that his son was in a complete remission—the minimal residual disease assessment was negative; however, he had not received sufficient anti-leukemia therapy to assure long-term survival and cure. I told him the risk of relapse with prolonged delays in therapy is real and not insignificant, but any perturbation, or depression of his immune system could be catastrophic and inhibit his ability to battle the pneumocystis infection. We waited, withheld chemotherapy, and prayed.

"I understand—*Baruch Hashem.*"

Harris' management was solely the province of the critical care team. The attendings, fellows, and residents rotated off service as their tenure on the unit changed weekly. Constancy and continuity of care was provided by Carol Vasquez, his bedside nurse, and Valerie Schocat, the physician assistant.

Most, if not all, of the body's vital functions were controlled by the myriad mechanical technology and pharmaceuticals to sustain life. The *whoosh, whoosh* of the respirator diaphragm as it bellowed up and down dictated the respiratory rate—the oxygen level was maintained by increasing the concentration of inspired gases. Heart function was maintained by ionotropic drugs to mitigate chances of failure, increase cardiac output, and prevent a buildup of fluids in his lungs. The recently started ECMO was working; his kidney and liver function were stable. Dr. Carroll was pleased with his progress.

The Pediatric Intensive Care Unit at Columbia occupies more than 50 beds on 2 floors, the 9th and 11th. Eleven Central is one of the few pediatric neurology and neurosurgery intensive care units in the country that is dedicated to patients with brain injury and disease. On the ninth floor, the Pediatric Intensive Care Unit stretches the length of three contiguous buildings—Tower, North, and Central. Nine North is the Milstein Neonatal-Infant Cardiac unit, a first-in-the-country specialized center equipped to care for post-heart surgery cases in patients less than one year of age; Nine Tower is the Cardiac Intensive Care Unit for older children and adolescents. Harris' room, 912, was on Nine Central, a general medical section for patients with acute and critical non-surgical illness; the unit, supported by the Wall Street bank, Morgan Stanley, has a spaceship motif. There are 16 patient rooms, 8 on the Broadway side and 8 that overlook a garden, the central core of the entire medical center. The rooms are large in order to accommodate the requisite equipment contained in a modern ICU, sliding glass doors enclose each room, and floor to ceiling curtains may be drawn for privacy. Outside each room is a desk and computer; in the center of the unit are the nursing station and a glass enclosed conference room for the physicians and staff to convene. Access to Nine Central is from the Tower or North Building with an elevator lobby on both sides.

Intensive care units are active 24 hours a day, 7 days a week. There is always a new critically ill patient from the operating room after major cardiac, liver, or brain surgery or a child with an acute asthmatic attack or diabetic ketoacidosis admitted through the emergency room. In addition, having a reputation as the best intensive care unit in the New York metropolitan area for children, a day never passes without the transfer of a case from an outside, referring hospital. It is a busy place. The lights are on and shine brightly all day and night; there are no clocks mounted on the walls—time doesn't matter. When patients need care, the staff and physicians provide it regardless of the hour. Fortunately, Harris was more than holding his own—not out of the danger, but in a good place.

On an early Friday morning while walking from my office on the seventh floor of the Irving Pavilion to Pediatric Grand Rounds in the amphitheater on the first floor of the Black Building, I made a detour to visit Harris. His overnight nurse, Rebecca Anthony, was at the computer, charting the relevant lab results and numbers.

"Good morning," I said, "Can you give me a quick clinical update? How was the night—anything I should know? Anything I can help you with?"

"No, he is quite stable. Everything is about the same."

I entered the room, pushed aside the privacy curtain, and opened the glass doors. Mr. Schulman was standing in the back corner of the room, his *tallith*, or prayer shawl, covering his head and *tefillin* on his forehead and wrapped around his left arm. *Tefillin* are cubic, black leather boxes with leather straps that men wear during weekday morning prayers—a daily ritual for observant Orthodox and Hasidic men. The boxes contain four handwritten texts from the Bible, in which believers are commanded to wear certain words on the hand and between the eyes. The texts are Exodus 13:1-10 and 13:11-16, and Deuteronomy 6:4-9 and 11:12-21. I did not disturb his trance-like incantations, but I was certain he sensed my presence in the room.

I walked to the head of the bed. Harris was motionless. Rebecca had recently given him his daily bath, washed him from head to toe, applied moisturizing cream to his body, and covered him with a clean sheet. He was ready to face a new day. Hopefully it would be a day similar to the previous day and the day before that.

I thought to myself, *Boring is a good thing for ICU patients.*

I touched his shoulder and his forehead. He was warm to the touch—an indication of life, though life sustained by medical intervention. I pondered the hypothetical: *If the respirator, renal dialysis, and ECMO were withdrawn, would he survive? Probably not.*

As I was about to leave the unit, Mr. Schulman completed his prayers and asked if he could ask me a question.

"Of course."

"Is it safe for me to leave for *Shabbos* and have dinner with my wife and other children? She's preparing matzah ball soup and brisket. Her parents are visiting from Monsey for the weekend. I've arranged for a volunteer from Chai Lifeline to be with Harris. What do you think?"

"Well, now would be a good time. Harris is stable. There is a good team on call for the weekend, but be certain to answer your cell phone if you see a number from the hospital—305 or 342—or my mobile phone, which I know you already have. Promise me."

"Absolutely. No worries. I'll answer my phone. I'll be back after *Shabbos,* Saturday night."

When I stopped by the ICU at the end of the day, Mr. Schulman had already left to be certain he was in Brooklyn before sundown—the tradition. I peeked into the room, Harris seemed to be the same—good lab values, stable vital signs. An uneventful day; a good omen for a quiet weekend. Alicia met me on Broadway and 165th Street in front of the children's hospital at 4 p.m. with Clementine, our tri-color Cavalier King Charles Spaniel, who was asleep on the back seat of the Audi Q5. Alicia put the flashing hazard lights on, moved to the passenger seat and I got into the driver's seat for the less than two-hour trip to our weekend retreat in Salisbury, Connecticut.

We had purchased the house on Ravine Ridge Road 10 years ago. It had previously been owned for more than 30 years by Sol Stein, a prominent New York attorney and Judaic scholar, and his wife, Edna, a philanthropist and board member at Sloan Kettering Memorial Hospital. Sol's collection of Jewish books and historical objects had occupied every bookshelf in every room; thousands of items that were donated to the New York Jewish Museum upon his death.

It was our special place—an almost 200-year-old barn-style sanctuary that we had renovated and modernized completely. There is a trout stream and waterfall on the property that separated the states of Connecticut and Massachusetts; we were the last house in Connecticut. Our house allowed us to restore our batteries and spend time together. Alicia tended to her vegetable garden, and I weeded and pruned the flowerbeds. We exercised. I played golf at Wyantenuck Country Club, and Alicia enjoyed the Farmers Market in Great Barrington and shopping at Guido's, the Big Y, and TJ Maxx. At night, we binge-watched *The Marvelous Mrs. Maisel* or *Ray Donovan*. Weekends at the house were close to perfect.

On Saturday morning, I called Danica Boyko, the fellow on call, to get an update on Harris. She indicated that he had a low-grade fever and blood cultures had been obtained and sent to the microbiology lab for analysis, but otherwise his condition was unchanged—lab values, chest x-ray, and blood gases were all stable. The ICU team decided not to begin broad-spectrum antibiotics but rather to continue observation. I agreed with the plan. I asked Danica to keep me updated.

Mr. Schulman returned to his son's bedside Sunday morning and participated in critical care rounds led by Dr. Beth Smith, the attending on call. He was frightened to learn that the fever persisted, unabated. Although the cultures obtained the day before had not yet yielded results, Beth decided to add Zosyn, piperacillin/tazobactam, as a precaution. Critically ill patients in intensive care units are at risk of infection secondary to the interventions and equipment needed to keep them alive; the risk is heightened in leukemic patients as they are immunosuppressed from the disease and its treatment, rendering them particularly vulnerable to bacterial sepsis.

Mr. Schulman called my mobile phone. "Dr. Weiner, what's happening?"

I told Mr. Schulman that I'd spoken to Drs. Smith and Danica Boyko. I told him that the Zosyn was routine, prophylactic; the cultures were negative so far and Harris remained quite stable. There was no cause for concern. I urged him to be calm and call again if he needed me, explaining that I would see him in the morning.

On Monday morning, I joined the ICU rounds as an observer. I was not on service but was concerned about Harris. The cast of characters changed— Beth Smith led the team. She is an experienced intensivist, triple-boarded in pediatrics, anesthesiology, and critical care medicine. We have known one another 40 years. I like her; she is easy to work with and never takes herself too seriously. Carol Vasquez, Valerie Schocat, and Mr. Schulman were waiting outside Room 912. The fellows and residents were new to the unit but quickly got up to speed and were well-versed in Harris' case.

There was a new finding: fever—now 103 degrees—and cultures positive for Staphylococcus aureus. Otherwise, the patient was stable and not dramatically different over the course of the last week to 10 days. His vital signs were stable, the blood gases and oxygen level satisfactory, chest x-ray unchanged, renal and liver function normal, and his complete blood count continued to be adequate without evidence of leukemia relapse. Beth had spoken to the infectious disease doctors, and they suggested continuing the Zosyn and adding Vancomycin; we all agreed.

Mr. Schulman asked, "Where did this come from? How did it happen? What is the significance? Will he survive?"

I allowed Beth Smith to answer. I would embellish if needed, but Harris was really under her care. She told him that Staphylococcus was not uncommon in ICU patients on respirators and ECMO who require multiple interventions, blood draws, and tests. She explained that, fortunately, Harris' white count is good—he was not neutropenic, and hopefully we could manage effectively with the antibiotics.

I added, "If he were neutropenic, I think our concern would be greater, but as long as he is stable and his counts remain good, he should weather this infection."

Mr. Schulman seemed relieved—concerned, but, for the moment, comfortable with the explanation. He retreated to the side of his son's bed, placed his left hand on his forehead, held his little black prayer book with his right hand, and prayed silently.

I was in clinic Wednesday morning when Beth Smith called my mobile phone. "Michael, I am worried about Harris. His fever is 104 degrees. He has a new skin rash and is neutropenic. His platelets dropped to 25,000, and his liver transaminases are rising. The sedimentation rate is 77 and CRP, 15. Initially, we thought the rash was secondary to the vancomycin, but putting everything together, we are concerned about HLH."

"Did you get triglycerides, fibrinogen, and ferritin levels?"

"Already drawn."

A diagnosis of HLH, hemophagocytic lymphohistiocytosis, would be disastrous. It would be difficult to treat and would diminish Harris' chance of survival. It is an unusual disorder of the immune system. The resultant cytokine storm, activation histiocytes, and T-cells as well as decreased NK (natural killer) cell function causes significant morbidity and mortality.

I was shocked and terrified. Harris had been stable, holding his own, and slowly improving from the pneumocystis infection. Now, disaster. His father would be crushed.

"Beth, I'm with a new patient. Give me an hour. I'd like to join you when you speak to Mr. Schulman. Let's draw a CD25, soluble IL 2 receptor. Should we send to a sample to Cincinnati for gene testing?"

"Yes, already done; I called Arush to join as well. Let's meet at noon."

Mr. Schulman, a keen observer, sensed something had gone awry. Harris' fever persisted, he had a yellowish hue to his skin from an elevated bilirubin level, and he developed petechiae, micro-skin hemorrhages secondary to a low platelet count.

The father was anxious, shaken, but not alone. A fraternity exists among the parents and families whose children are in the intensive care unit. Although each child is in a single room, the physical structure of the unit is open—a "safety in numbers" mentality exists. The families support one another—well wishes, prayers, food from home, errands, offers to help in any way. When a child takes a turn, everyone is aware. Coming to Mr. Joseph's aid was the African-American mother of a son with sickle cell anemia who had acute chest syndrome, the Muslim father of a teenage boy with a ruptured spleen from an automobile accident, and the Chinese parents of an infant girl with cystic fibrosis and an overwhelming pulmonary infection. There are no barriers where critically ill children are concerned; race, language, cultural disparity do not exist; families help each other. Privacy was respected but was difficult to maintain. Collectively, they offered prayers and healing thoughts.

Beth Smith, Arush Krishana, and I met with Mr. Schulman in the small conference room just off the elevator lobby. Arush is one of the stem cell transplant and cellular therapies attendings. He has particular expertise in

HLH, which he developed due to the fact that his transplant patients have an increased incidence of the disease. Arush's parents fled Pakistan in the 1970s and settled in Bhopal, India. His family lived in abject poverty; his parents and five children occupied a small house—perhaps 100 square feet that they shared with his father's cows. Each morning, Arush went door-to-door, delivering milk in the slum-like neighborhood. He was the first in his family to attend high school and college, working in a pharmacy dispensing medicine after school to offset educational expenses. His mother wanted him to become a doctor, a career path which solidified as he observed Ramesh, a younger brother, die from acute myelogenous leukemia without receiving appropriate treatment. After medical school in India, Arush completed a pediatric residency at The Brooklyn Hospital Center and a fellowship in pediatric hematology-oncology and stem cell transplant at the University of South Carolina and Columbia. He joined the transplant and cellular therapy faculty in 2005 and has remained an incredible teacher, physician, and colleague.

During our meeting, Mr. Schulman appeared, ashen and clearly shaken by the downturn in his son's condition. Arush explained our concern about HLH and explained the extreme gravity of the condition, indicating that the mortality was high. He recommended high dose steroids and etoposide, a chemotherapy drug with specificity against the cytokine storm of HLH.

Mr. Schulman, perplexed, asked, "Won't the steroids make treating infections more difficult? Can he survive? Are you doing everything for him? I'm scared."

For the very first time, I expressed concern. I was worried; we were all worried. Harris faced two life-threatening infections—pneumocystis in his lungs and Staph. aureus in the blood—and had seemed to weather the storm. But now he was pancytopenic, bleeding, and to add insult to injury, HLH; it might be more than he could overcome and survive. Beth Smith told Mr. Schulman that the critical care team was completely committed to life and would spare nothing and employ every medical resource available.

Beth said, "We will continue the antibiotics, respirator, ECMO, and dialysis, will transfuse blood and platelets as needed, monitor every organ system function, and deal with the HLH as best as we can. You have my word."

"Baruch Hashem."

As we left the conference room, the elevator door opened and nine Hasidic men dressed in black, several appearing younger than Harris, stepped into the lobby. Speaking in Yiddish, the oldest among them told Mr. Schulman that they were here to pray with him. Mr. Schulman and group of strangers retreated to the *minyan* room, a small sparse room with a faux altar and 10 chairs on the eighth floor that New York Presbyterian Hospital had established to accommodate the religious needs of the Jewish orthodox families whose children received care at Columbia. In Judaism, a *minyan* is the quorum of 10 Jewish adult men required for certain religious obligations. Together, they recited the *"Mi Shebeirach,"* a beautiful, lyrical prayer dedicated to friends or loved ones who are struggling with physical, emotional, or spiritual challenges—the prayer speaks to healing and peace.

What more could be done? Time and prayer seemed appropriate and best. I had every confidence that if Harris was meant to survive, he would. Dr. Smith and the PICU team would do everything conceivable, spare no modality, leave no stone uncovered, but frankly, survival was in God's hands. I knew it, Mr. Schulman knew it, Beth Smith knew it, the residents, fellows, nurses knew it, and the other parents knew it.

As I left Nine Central, I was sick to my stomach. My head was replete with a multitude of emotions and thoughts, not the least of which was bona fide deep-seated thoughts of Harris' death. I thought about Mr. Schulman and how he had buried a wife and so many family members; how could he endure the death of a son? I thought about my career and how in the 1970s and '80s, death was common in children with cancer. I thought about how often I would be in the hospital in the middle of the night trying to comfort a family whose son or daughter had just died. Frankly, there were no words of condolence to ease their grief and pain. I thought about how parents would thank me for all that I had done on behalf of their child; how odd . . . their son or daughter had just died, and I let them down. *Don't thank me.*

I had another thought—this of the expense of keeping Harris and patients like him alive. The resources required to sustain life—ECMO, dialysis, ventilators, antibiotics, blood work, x-rays . . . the list is endless and costly. Hospital intensive care unit expenditures exceed $4,500 per day plus professional fees for physicians. A back of the envelope estimate exceeds half a million dollars. What is the value a life? An unanswerable question.

We were back at square one. The small gains achieved were erased; the monotonous rhythm of sameness evolved to chaos. Leukemia, pneumocystis, staph sepsis, multiple organ failure all seemed trivial; HLH would be a formidable foe. Victory would be a hard-fought confrontation measured by small, incremental battles. Survival would take everything we had—knowledge, diligence, technology, and most importantly, great nurses. Thankfully, I believe we had the tools to prevail.

As I walked back to clinic, I asked God for his help—*let Harris live.*

Three days passed. The serum markers for HLH, ferritin, and CRP, although remarkably elevated, had stopped rising and stabilized. Harris' chest x-ray continued to improve, though slowly; his blood cultures, previously positive for staph, had reverted to negative. Hepatic, renal, respiratory, and cardiac functions all inching positively towards recovery. The high dose steroids, etoposide, supportive measures, and the incomparable bedside care were beginning to show dividends.

Mr. Schulman called my cell phone and asked if I would come to the PICU at 3 p.m., "I want to introduce you to someone."

"Yes, of course."

"Dr. Weiner, this is Rachel, my new wife."

"Pleasure to meet you, Rachel."

Rachel seemed atypical for a Hasidic woman, more modern; she wore a *sheitel*, the Yiddish term for a wig, but her stylish dark-blue dress, matching shoes, and a pearl necklace belied her Hasidic routes.

Rachel greeted me warmly but, as was the custom, we did not shake hands, rather simply acknowledging one another.

I detected a glimmer of a smile on Mr. Schulman's face. He was most assuredly more relaxed responding to Harris' progress.

"Doctor, could it be true? Dr. Smith told us this morning that she is pleased. She had guarded optimism."

My judgment and experience necessitated a reality check. Harris remained on ECMO, was still respirator dependent, and manifested persistent evidence of organ failure and inflammation secondary to HLH. But was he better? Yes. Still, we had been down this road before only to be disappointed by a new problem or complication from illness or treatment. I tried to temper his enthusiasm without dampening his excitement; I walked a fine line, a path taken frequently when communicating with parents of children with cancer, especially in the critical care unit.

I reverted to, "Mr. Schulman, there is no question that Harris seems more stable and, by every assessment, he is again on an upward trajectory. If it is God's will, he will survive."

"Baruch Hashem."

My cell phone rang, and the caller ID identified Dr. Bill Simons, my mother's internist in Florida. "Michael, I am with Lucille in the emergency room at JFK Hospital. She doesn't look good. I think you should come to Florida as soon as you can."

Bill Simon's call did not come as a surprise. I had been expecting it—if not that day, soon . . . very soon. The thought of death terrified my mother, terrified my sister Margaret, terrified me. I spoke to Lucille every evening as I drove home from Columbia. "Hi Mom, how are you today?"

"Okay," she'd mumble. "I love you."

"I love you too, Mom. I'll speak to you tomorrow."

It became apparent that with each passing hour, day, week, month, she was readying herself to die. Still, I was not prepared. I still needed her in my life. Not her spirit and blessed memory, but *her* in the flesh—her smile, her smell, her touch, her gargled voice. We all knew Lucille's path mapped to her worldly departure, but she was my mother. I was heartbroken and not accepting of her death.

I told Mr. Schulman that something had come up that necessitated my absence from the hospital for a few days. I mentioned that I'd check in and said that if needed, I could be reached at any time of the day or night on my cell. He knew that the intensive care doctors were excellent and had confidence in Paul Thomas, the doctor on service after Dr. Smith. I told him, "Your son will be in my prayers."

I shook hands with Mr. Schulman and said goodbye to Rachel. I did not tell them the reason for my impromptu departure.

"Well, enjoy your time away."

As I walked back to clinic, I asked God for his help—*let Harris live*—and added a prayer for restful peace for my mother.

Alicia and I abruptly made arrangements to travel to Lake Worth, Florida to be with my 98-year-old mother for the last time.

She lived in The Fountains, a sprawling playground of activities for snow-birds from New York, Chicago, and Toronto. My parents, Bill and Lucille, bought a house on Fountains Circle Drive over 25 years ago. It was quite nice actually. My mom was an exceptional interior designer in her day— she decorated their two-bedroom, two-and-a-half-bath home beautifully in all beige. Everything was beige. The walls, floors, rugs, sofas, chairs, armoires, and artwork—beige. And anything that wasn't beige was glass and mirrors. It worked.

When my dad passed away six years prior, my sister, Margaret, and I wanted Lucille to sell the house in Florida and return to New York to be near children, grandchildren, and great-grandchildren. She refused. She had a life at The Fountains—independent, attractive for 92, and her sister, Rosa Lee, lived in Boca Raton, two towns away. She played bridge, canasta, drove her beige Mercedes-Benz, and had a group of friends, both men and women. She was staying—no discussion.

Lucille had a gentleman friend—a widower—Arnie Katz. They had known one another for years and were friends and companions. One evening, as Lucille prepared for a dinner date with Arnie at The Fountains Country Club, the phone rang. In her haste to answer the call, she slipped on the kitchen floor and fractured her right hip and femur. Instead of dinner, she spent the night in the emergency room of JFK Hospital on Congress Boulevard. She needed emergency surgery to save her leg and stop the hemorrhaging. A rod was inserted into the entire length of her femur, from the pelvis to her knee. Recovery and rehabilitation subsequent to such injury is difficult at any age, but at 92, it borders on impossible. My mother's life would never be the same; however, she continued to refuse to leave Florida and move back to New York.

After the injury, Lucille was different. Her physical condition necessitated a full-time, live-in nurse's aide. Enter Mary Codner, an affable Jamaican woman whose family lived in Port St. Lucie. Mary's husband, a long-distance truck driver, was frequently on the road and her two boys were married and had their own families. She affectionately called my mother Lucy Lu; she was a blessing, physically strong, cared deeply for my mother, and the situation allowed her to remain in her own home.

Lucy Lu's condition deteriorated. She devolved from walker to wheelchair, to total dependency on Mary, who moved her from her bed, to the kitchen table, to her chair in the den, to the kitchen table, to her bed. She left her house only for doctor appointments and the weekly trip to Costco for adult diapers, Ensure, and paper towels. She either would not or could not eat or take sips of water, and her breathing became labored. Mary managed to get her in the car and drove to the JFK Emergency Room. Bill Simons did a cursory assessment and called me on my cell phone.

Alicia and I were on a JetBlue flight from Westchester to West Palm Beach International the next morning. Margaret arrived from LaGuardia on a Delta flight, and we met her in my mom's room, 2106. Mary was there as well. Though Lucille had survived the night, death was near; that was obvious.

While in Florida, I was too preoccupied with Lucille to read Harris' daily progress notes, but Beth Smith sent an email: blood results, CBC, indicators of liver, renal function, inflammatory markers of HLH—normal; chest x-ray—dramatically improved. He was extubated, removed from the respirator, and ECMO was terminated.

I thanked God for his help—Harris would survive. Lucille would not.

I received a text message on my mobile phone from Mr. Schulman, telling me his prayers had been answered.

Harris Schulman's life is a testament to the merger of medical technology, determination, and prayer.

Baruch Hashem.

Harris remained in the ICU for several more days before he could be safely transferred to Tower 5. But he made it; he would live. That *Shabbos*, Mr. Schulman joined Rachel and family in Brooklyn. He davened Saturday morning at his *shul* in Williamsburg, read from the Torah—the Hebrew book of laws and prayers—and enjoyed *kiddush*, wine, and food with friends and neighbors. The entire community was elated, overjoyed; their prayers were answered.

I loved my mother, as did Margaret, Alicia, the grandchildren, and great-grandchildren. She was a beautiful, elegant woman. I knew her time was near, but I was not ready to say goodbye.

Room 2106 was nondescript. It was filled with three chairs, a TV mounted on the pale gray wall, windows overlooking the parking lot, and my precious mom, lying in the bed in the center of the room. Moaning and agitated, she mumbled, "Help me up; help me up."

I leaned close to her left ear and, with tears beginning to well up, I whispered, "I love you, Mom."

Our eyes were transfixed on the monitor displaying pulse rate and oxygen saturation. The readings were not accurate—of that I was certain—not that it mattered one iota. She was agitated and restless. Her eyes were closed, her mouth open. Her death was near.

I called Dr. Simon and suggested that he order a small dose of Ativan to lessen her struggle to breathe. We discussed hospice care to allow her to die at home, and he agreed. Ativan 0.5 mg IV worked effectively; she relaxed and was calm for the moment. My mother did not look like my mother. She more closely resembled a skeletal Auschwitz survivor with her sunken eyes, extreme pallor, skin marred with bruises, and weeping sores. Yet, when Margaret asked her if she was in any pain, she indicated no.

On Sunday morning, we met Lila Taggert, the Trust Bridge hospice coordinator. Lila was raised in Teaneck, New Jersey, and her father lived at The Fountains and drove a dark blue Bentley convertible. She wore a white coat and leopard print Michael Kors shoes. She was an attentive, competent, no-nonsense nurse who possessed a special talent for cutting through red tape and expediting the needed complexities of transferring Lucille to her home. A hospital bed, oxygen, medications, and supplies were delivered to 6815 Fountains Circle at 4 p.m., and the ambulance arrived at JFK at 6 o'clock. The EMTs respectfully and carefully wrapped Lucille in blankets, placed her on the stretcher, and transported her to the waiting medical van for the short ride home.

Gigi, the hospice nurse, had everything prepared for Lucille's arrival. The hospital bed was in the beige living room. The EMTs gently placed her in bed. She recognized immediately that she was home and asked to sit in her black reclining chair in the den. Mary carried her to the den with as much care as if she had been a treasured, priceless heirloom. Lucille smiled and seemed to whisper, "Thank you."

As Gigi gently fed Lucille some soft vanilla ice cream, she toyed with the coolness on her lips. *60 Minutes* was playing on the TV, but no one was watching. After an hour, Mary placed her back in the hospital bed. She was agitated, restless. Gigi administered a small dose of Ativan subcutaneously, followed by Roxanol, oral morphine drops, on her tongue. Thankfully, she relaxed and fell asleep. Breathing was difficult and came in ineffective gasps with her mouth open. We expected that night to be her last. Alicia, Margaret, Mary, and I alternated bedside vigilance. She survived the night.

Amy replaced Gigi on Monday morning. She was young, had tattoos on her arms, and was soft-spoken, caring, and respectful of what was unfolding. Margaret and I held our mom's head in our grasp, caressed her forehead, kissed her cheeks, and told her that we loved her and that it was okay to die. She needed our permission, and we reluctantly offered our consent. Her breaths were intermittent, her heart rate slowed. Lucille passed away peacefully with Margaret, Alicia, and me at her side. We cried as we held our mom and each other. We loved our mother so. Our beautiful, sacrificing mother was gone—at peace.

The funeral, at Eternal Light Cemetery in Boynton Beach, was Wednesday afternoon. There was no fanfare; just our small family, children, and grandchildren, Lucille's sister Rosa Lee, cousins Marilyn, Mogens, and their son, Jonah. We stopped at the Beth Israel funeral home before the cemetery to say one last goodbye. The beige casket was open. Mom, dressed in a beige suit, was cold, lifeless, and hard.

"Come on, Mom. Get up. Talk to me. I love you, Mom. Don't go."

I was not prepared. I anticipated Lucille's death; expected it. If not today, tomorrow, next week, next month. It was imminent. Yet, I was not prepared; Margaret was not prepared; Alicia was not prepared; the grandchildren were not prepared.

The service was brief. Rabbi Marc Lebowitz respected our wishes, offering a short prayer, the 23rd Psalm, and the Mourner's Kaddish. Margaret told us about her lifelong love for Lucille, and I chokingly read a simple poem.

> Flowers grow in Heaven
>   Of that I have no doubt
> I picked a bunch for my mother
>   And told her they're from me
> I told my Mom I love her
>   I gave her a tender kiss for all to see
> Remembering my Mom is easy
>   I'll speak with her every day
> But there will always be an empty feeling
>   That will never go away

Together we placed the casket in a mausoleum with her head adjacent to my father, William.

"Goodbye, Mom. I love you."

I returned to Columbia the following Monday morning after nine days of radio silence. There had not been a word about Harris. I assumed no news to be good news. I searched the list of inpatients, but his name was conspicuously absent.

He had been discharged the previous Friday before *Shabbos*, for dinner at home with family—chicken matzah ball soup and brisket; how great is that? At *shul* on Saturday morning, the congregation cheered his presence. My goodness, Harris had survived pneumocystis, staph sepsis, HLH, and multiple organ failure. Perhaps it was a miracle, but it assuredly was also a triumph of the human spirit and resilience.

Harris, accompanied by Mr. Schulman, came to clinic on Tuesday. I was elated to see them both. Harris had lost 30 pounds and was extremely deconditioned but alive. He had not received leukemia treatment in almost two months. His blood counts were excellent. I performed a bone marrow aspirate to assess his status, and remarkably, his MRD test was negative; there was no evidence of leukemia—complete remission.

I asked Harris if he had any memory of what had transpired and of how sick he had been. He told me that he did not, but his father had related what he had unknowingly experienced. I explained to Harris that he required a year of maintenance therapy, which would be all outpatient, weekly visits. I urged him to be diligent about taking his Bactrim.

"Don't worry about that, Dr. Weiner."

He told me that he was going to enroll in an EMT course and volunteer for the local Hatzolah Emergency Medical Service.

"That's a great idea!"

"Dr. Weiner, do you think I could go medical school and become a doctor?"

MICHAEL WEINER

Columbia Presbyterian

There was something unique about James Bergen's hands—big, soft, reassuring.

James had just been appointed Chairman of the Department of Pediatrics at the Babies Hospital at Columbia Presbyterian Medical Center, and we were discussing my recruitment as the Director of the Division of Pediatric Oncology. James was a big man; he had an affable smile, prominent facial features, and a congenial personality. He'd spent his career in the nursery, caring for critically ill newborns, and I often wondered how he managed to do procedures on premature infants that weighed barely more than a pound. But he did. He was an excellent physician and an extraordinary teacher, having trained a generation of neonatologists. He was revered and adored by parents, and all who knew him. James was iconic.

It was a beautiful, early summer day, and we met in the dining room of my home on Woodhill Road in Tenafly, New Jersey. Sitting in high-backed, mauve mohair chairs, we spread papers and notes on the art deco, black lacquer table. The room had a circular windowed alcove that overlooked the backyard, and the perennials were in full bloom. Alicia greeted James warmly, served coffee and croissants, and told us she was leaving for work in the city. Lauren and Eli were at camp.

James told me that he wanted me to return to Babies Hospital and rebuild the child cancer program. He said that with Luigi Scarletta as director, the program had suffered greatly and needed work, and he believed I was the right man for the job. I knew immediately that my answer was yes. I knew Luigi, had worked with him in the past. He sported a ponytail atop his balding head; it was a look. In fairness, Luigi was an outstanding hematologist, trained at Harvard, made major contributory discoveries in the field of red blood cell enzymes, thalassemia, and lead poisoning, but he cared little about children with cancer.

James asked me if I was interested in returning to Columbia and what I required as a recruitment package; the number of physicians I'd need, my thoughts about a research enterprise, administrative needs, office space, clinical space, academic rank, salary, an endowed chair—the list was long.

He asked, "How many new patients do you think you will see in the first year, second year, third year? We need to be certain that the hospital ramps up appropriately to accommodate a growing program."

Frankly, I had no idea. There was a risk. I knew it, and James knew it. I did not want to be overly aggressive in estimating new patient volume, but I did not want to be conservative, as it could lead to reduced services. "Well, I think 50 new patients in year one is realistic and perhaps 100 cases by year three."

James and I were both new at this game. The person doing the recruitment doesn't want to offer an oversized package, whereas the person being recruited always wants more than is being offered, at least initially. Fortunately, we were honest friends and mostly wanted the same thing: to restore the pediatric cancer program to prominence. We easily reached an agreement. I would be offered an endowed chair, I would be the Hettinger Professor of Pediatrics, Director of Pediatric Oncology at the Babies Hospital and Columbia University College of Physicians and Surgeons—my start date: January 1, 1997. This was an honor, a big step forward in my career, and frankly, I was humbled.

I prioritized two immediate goals. The first was to build a referral base to attract patients, and the second was finding extraordinary people to join us on this journey.

I met Arthur Schwartz for breakfast at Shalom, a kosher restaurant on the Upper West Side of Manhattan. Despite my aversion to kosher anything, I made an exception for Arthur who was great, a talented solid-tumor specialist and clinical investigator. He graduated from Boston University's six-year combined bachelor's and medical doctor program, served as a house office at Albert Einstein, and had been at the National Cancer Institute in Bethesda as a fellow and attending. I offered Arthur a position on the spot as the Associate Director. He accepted.

Together, we met Cora Kenny, a graduating fellow from CHOP, the Children's Hospital of Philadelphia. Cora had an impeccable resume, but equally important, we knew her personally, liked her, and felt that she would be a good fit for us. Cora became a close friend. She was one of the most intelligent and hardest-working physicians I have ever had the privilege of working with and I learned something new from her every day.

A search for a researcher led us to Daniel Hito, an MD, PhD from New York University who was Cora's colleague at CHOP. He studied molecular pathways in neuroblastoma with Gary Barrett, who gave him high marks, and told us Daniel had great potential for success. I had a gut feeling about Daniel and offered him a job at Columbia, which he accepted. My gut was correct, Daniel has had a terrific career.

Arthur, Cora, Daniel, and I formed the nucleus of our new division; we inherited Thomas Klavrock and James Moore, two holdovers from the previous administration. Klavrock, an elf-like figure, was my contemporary. We were certain he was on the autism spectrum—probably Asperger's syndrome. He had an MD, PhD from Jefferson in Philadelphia and had trained as a resident and fellow at Boston Children's and Dana-Farber Cancer Institute. His knowledge base was expansive, he had a photographic memory, forgot nothing, and kept records on everything. His office file cabinets stood from floor to ceiling, with stacks of papers occupying every square inch of space. It was hard to open the door to the office because of clutter, and he sat at a desk totally obscured from view, essentially invisible. But despite these personal quirks, Klavrock was smart, and he took care of children with brain tumors so there would be a place for him in the division.

James Moore had no qualities that I admired. He was just fair as a physician caregiver, but for now, we needed a warm body; he would soon be history and would move on to another position.

As director of the division, I worked to develop key elements to my leadership style; I always put the careers of my colleagues first, and I never, *never* asked anyone to do anything I would not do myself. These simple rules served everyone well.

St. Joseph's Medical Center in Paterson, New Jersey, Valley Hospital in Ridgewood, New Jersey, Nyack Hospital in Nyack, New York, Winthrop Medical Center in Mineola, New York, Stanford Medical Center in Stanford, Connecticut, and Methodist Hospital in Brooklyn, New York were all on the hit list. I had personal relationships with key people at each institution, either the chief executive or the chair of pediatrics. In addition, Columbia Presbyterian had a number of affiliates, Harlem Hospital, Lincoln Hospital, and St. Luke's-Roosevelt, that were also in play. I created a medical service agreement at each institution that paid the division a fee to render care to patients in the community. The agreements stated that if the child had cancer, they would be transferred to the Babies Hospital, but for other consultations and problems, we'd manage them at the home hospital. This paradigm worked beautifully; it added revenue to the division bottom line and increased significantly the number of new patients at Babies with cancer. There was one caveat—everyone had to spend time at a community hospital, good and bad. I went to St. Joseph's and Valley Hospital, Cora Kenny to Nyack, Moore to Lincoln and Harlem. This became a real pain in the butt, but the strategy worked. The division treated more than 75 new patients in the first year and over 100 in year two. Importantly, we were finally financially solvent. James Bergen, Martin Long, the Chief Executive Officer of Columbia Presbyterian, and Marcus Fishland, the Dean of the medical school, were ecstatic; they thought I was the best thing since sliced bread. Of course, it was less me than the hard work of my colleagues, good decision making, great recruitments, and the ability to see opportunity as the magic sauce.

But this was about to change.

James Bergen and I were talking in his office on the first floor of the Babies Hospital. The office was nondescript—large desk, comfortable swivel chair, bookshelves, and a table and chairs for six. We were sitting at the table when the door flew open, and David Sklar, Chair of Pathology and a powerful presence at the medical center, stormed in, yelling, "Fire that fucking guy immediately. Today. Or pay the consequences; I mean it."

"David, calm down."

"Bergen, don't tell me to calm down, I'm serious. Get rid of that asshole. I got nothing else to say. No discussion."

Sklar slammed the door shut as abruptly as he'd jerked it open. James and I were dumbfounded; we learned that Arthur Schwartz was on call for the weekend and wanted to administer a white blood cell transfusion to a patient. The blood bank director told him, "Not possible."

Arthur called David Sklar directly, complaining that he was the attending on service and his patient needed granulocytes. Arthur told him that Columbia was a bush-league hospital; Sklar, not known for his ability to remain calm under the best of circumstances, wanted to cut Schwartz's balls off on the spot. Red-headed and -tempered, Arthur, never one to back down from a good argument, particularly one in which he felt he held the moral high ground, continued to berate Sklar, his blood bank, and his department. Schwartz's patient never received the white cells, and Bergen and I had to speak with Arthur.

We gave him a few days to cool off, and then Arthur and I spoke.

"Arthur, my *boychik*, what did you do? Sklar is outraged."

Arthur told me not to worry. He realized that Columbia was not a good place for him, and he had already accepted a position at Memorial Sloan Kettering. He would be leaving soon.

Personally, I adored Arthur. He was a terrific doctor, but he had an explosive temper. The situation with Sklar placed me in the untenable predicament of trying to both support and defend my faculty while simultaneously trying to mediate a solution or face the wrath of the Chair of Pathology. I like to believe that the former was possible, but Arthur had alleviated my burden and made my choice a non-decision.

On paper, Philip London was a superstar. His presentation was odd—standing up straight he was barely 5-feet, 2- or possibly 3-inches, with short arms and legs, and wild, mad professor hair, but his intellect was superior. His interests included developmental therapeutics, lymphoma, and stem cell transplant. He built a pediatric oncology program at Children's Hospital of Orange County, California, created the Pediatric Cancer Research Foundation, which supported his laboratory, and was now teaching at Georgetown in Washington, D.C. He was regarded internationally as a clinical investigator, but he also had a reputation as a manipulating narcissist.

Our division lacked a stem cell transplant program and a developmental-therapeutics program—two mandatory initiatives required to elevate the division and make us competitive, both in New York City and nationally. Enter Philip London. Daniel and Cora were both opposed and several colleagues, including Arthur Ballins, a former co-worker of London's in California, cautioned me against hiring him; everyone told me, "Don't do it!" I rationalized that I could get along with anyone, so why not London? James Bergen called his counterpart at Georgetown, who told us London was great—a flat out lie. He just wanted the stain removed from his department. We hired him, and he arrived at Columbia in March. By April, I was incredulous. It was an unmitigated disaster.

London had a contingent of loyalists. Three nurse practitioners and an administrator represented the core of his team. Two of the three, Lauren and Meghan, lived in southern California, but he insisted they have Columbia University appointments, despite living 3,000 miles away. He paid them from his personal Pediatric Cancer Research Foundation slush fund. His loyalists were indispensable; they wrote his papers, grant applications, and meeting abstracts. I questioned whether they wiped his ass after every bowel movement.

Several times a week, London sent an email blast to Bergen, Anne Hodges, the Director of the Columbia Cancer Center, other division directors, and hospital and university leadership, announcing that he had a paper accepted in a journal and a speaking engagement at some bullshit conference, or had been asked to give grand rounds at an obscure department of pediatrics in Podunk. No one had ever witnessed such unbelievable self-aggrandizement. His egotistical narcissism was like nothing I had ever experienced previously.

What's more, his leadership of the bone marrow transplant program was suspect. He selected patients for transplant that Sloan Kettering, CHOP, and Boston Children's refused because they had little chance of survival; his outcomes were terrible, he occupied beds unnecessarily, with high-risk patients remaining in the hospital for months, costing the hospital hundreds of thousands of dollars. The transplant program was hemorrhaging money and running a divisional deficit.

He lobbied Ellen Stein, Executive Director of the Babies Hospital, to create a separate division of stem cell transplant, and she relented. Ellen was a force of nature; a large woman, with coarse features and bouffant blond hair, she was an exceptional administrator. She had an obsequious manner but was never reluctant to trample and disrespect anyone in her way. She manhandled James Bergen and used Charles Fowler, former Chief of Pediatric Surgery, who gravitated to an administrative position as her punching bag. But she liked London.

Charles and I were friends and had been for more than 30 years. Charles likes to tell the story about when he first joined the Columbia faculty in the early 1980s, that I referred him his first surgical case, a teenage boy who needed a lymph node biopsy. Charles and I enjoyed playing golf together and during the summer we often stole a few hours late on a Thursday afternoon to play a quick 18 holes. Charles had an introduction to Hal Greene, an architect from Philadelphia whose firm was hired to do some work at the hospital. Greene happened to be a member at Pine Valley, perhaps the most exclusive golf club in the country and certainly the most difficult to join or even to play as a guest. Hal arranged for Charles and me to play at Pine Valley. I was more than ecstatic, however, he wanted to practice first, improve his game; so we waited. Two weeks before our scheduled round, the architectural firm was relieved of their responsibilities, Greene was incensed, blamed Charles, and we never got the chance to play. I will never forgive him.

Shortly thereafter, Charles retired from the hospital and Columbia, took the Series 7 exam, also known as the General Securities Representative Exam, to become qualified to purchase and/or sell security products such as stocks and bonds. He was going to join his son as a trader when he was diagnosed with severe, rapidly progressing Parkinson's disease and tragically died a dehumanizing death shortly thereafter. Horrible really.

London lacked honesty and academic integrity. I recall reading a paper regarding results on transplant patients undergoing tandem stem cell transplants for recurrent lymphoma. The lead author was Enrique Caballo, brother of Luis, the Academy Award-winning actor. After reading the manuscript, I questioned Enrique about the results, and he told me that he did not write the paper, had no idea about the study, the patients, or the results. Typical London; he was, of course, senior author on the manuscript that was undoubtedly written by his California girls.

The development therapeutics program always resides within oncology, but London attempted to commandeer the enterprise as his own. I bitterly resisted; I wanted a young person in our division to manage the program. He pushed back, and I fought harder. We were at each other's throats. Not only could we not be in the same room, we could not be on the same floor or in the same building.

As a result of his poor management, the transplant program ran a several hundred thousand dollar deficit. Bergen asked me to help.

"You're kidding. Absolutely not."

"Michael, I need you to be a good citizen of the department. It's important that Pediatrics, as a whole, be in the black. Divisions like oncology and neonatology that have the financial wherewithal must help support others for the good of the enterprise."

"James, I can't do it."

"Look, I am not asking you—I am telling you. I need 300 a year for three years."

"What? That is outrageous!"

"Michael, no more. Just do it!"

I disliked London more than any person I have ever interacted with. I contacted my friend James Doniva, the father of a former patient. James was from the old neighborhood, Little Italy, and he knew who to call to get certain things done. I thought about slashing London's tires or roughing him up a little—comical really. When I mentioned the predicament to James, he laughed at me and said, "Don't be ridiculous."

The relationship—or non-relationship—had become toxic and was affecting other members of the divisional faculty. Bergen insisted that London and I begin psychotherapy with a senior member of the Department of Psychiatry; there was no alternative but to agree.

Dr. Fisher's office was on 68th Street on the ground floor of an iconic westside building, steps from Central Park West. We met on Tuesdays at 8 a.m. The office had a small waiting room, but there was such rancor between us we would not sit in the anteroom together; the one who arrived second waited in the street for the session to begin. The office was large, comfortable, and decorated with a lifetime of Dr. Fisher's personal effects and artwork. There was a working fireplace, soft lighting, an antique desk, and a seating area with a sofa and four comfortable chairs. As Fisher introduced himself, London and I sat across from each other.

My blood was boiling. I had heart palpitations and could feel my blood pressure rising. What an uncomfortable sensation. We each spoke, and the anger was deep, tangible, and permeating. We accomplished little progress in resolving our differences and, if anything, the chasm between us deepened. He raised his voice, I spoke louder. I interrupted him, and he did the same to me. Dr. Fisher couldn't believe the anger and discord. Fisher told Bergen that we were not making progress—there was no middle ground, and we were all wasting time and money.

I have no doubt that, had we been a married couple, Dr. Fisher would proclaim that our differences mandated divorce with no hope of reconciliation. I was so pissed. My dislike for the guy had no boundaries.

Nothing changed.

Our cancer program grew, so we recruited additional faculty. All had exceptional pedigrees—Ivy League-educated, impeccable curriculum vitaes—but the *sine qua non* was that I feel a personal trust and connection with each individual, and trust on an emotional level that they would be a good fit for the division. Jacki Blade Gender and Margarita Robles from Memorial Sloan Kettering were two such examples.

I liked Jacki from the first time I met her. Her resume was extraordinary, having graduated from Yale University and Penn, her intelligence was a given, and barring some unforeseen crisis, it was clear that JBG would have an awesome career.

Margarita was educated at Columbia and Harvard, spoke five languages, and was an accomplished violinist and true renaissance individual. Her issue was that she was diffuse, lacked focus, and, in my judgement, never reached her full potential. A jack of all trades, but a master of none.

In order to enhance our research enterprise, we recruited Carlos Herrnando, an MD, PhD from Harvard. His mentor, Bob Shine, told me that Carlos was the single best scientist he had ever trained, so hiring him was an easy decision. Two obstacles remained, though—space and money. Antonio Delavra, Head of the Institute of Cancer Genetics and Director of the Irving Comprehensive Cancer Center and a world-renown cancer researcher, provided laboratory space and access to core resources. Hope & Heroes provided a million-dollar recruitment package for salary, personnel, and equipment. He continues to be a brilliant investigator studying childhood leukemia. An Bo Chang and Lucia Formigio joined from Harvard and Albert Einstein respectively. An's research involved bone marrow failure, and Lucia studied brain tumors. Delavra provided laboratory space and core resources and our foundation start-up financial support; a powerful partnership. Their research output has been at such a high level that both are tenured professors at Columbia University—not an easy accomplishment.

I recognized that the financial stability of the oncology program resided in philanthropy. The traditional revenue streams, patient income, hospital funds for delivered service, and research grants fell far short of the revenue needed to support the enterprise. It was this environment from which I founded an independent 501(c)(3), Hope & Heroes Children's Cancer Fund.

Hope & Heroes is a phenomenon that began in a backroom from a few phone calls to friends and family. A phenomenon that embraced a commitment to ease the pain and suffering of children with cancer. A phenomenon that has raised close to $100 million, supports 40 percent of the annual budget of the division, and provides resources for patient and family needs including rent, utilities, medications, and transportation. A phenomenon that provides integrative therapies, survivor wellness programs, and psychosocial care, while enabling the developmental therapeutics program. A phenomenon that facilitates faculty retention, new faculty recruitment, and educational post-doctoral training for the fellowship program. A phenomenon that funds the operating budget with current-use dollars and endowed chairs that recognize and honor donors with gifts in perpetuity. A phenomenon that has raised $2.5 million for each of four endowed chairs. The chief of the division is the Herb and Kayla Roberts Endowed Professor, and upon my retirement, there will be two Michael Weiner, MD endowed professorships for key faculty.

Colleagues around the country recognized Columbia as a pediatric oncology program of excellence. By every measure, we excelled, from patient care to research and education, and we were financially solvent. Our *U.S. News & World Report* ranking reached number 15, whereas eight years prior we had been virtually unknown.

One evening in the fall of 2006, Bergen landed in the ICU. He had left the hospital alone, crossed Broadway, and been hit by a car. The driver did not stop. An ambulance arrived and took him to the emergency department on 168th Street, less than half a block away from the accident. James sustained multiple internal injuries, a punctured lung, and required several surgeries. He was lucky to be alive. It took six months before he was able to return to work, but he was not the same. He was physically slower, and mentally he was no match for our executive director, Ellen Stein, and was unable to represent the interests of the Department of Pediatrics. In 2008, about two years after the accident, he announced his retirement.

It took more than a year to recruit the new chair, Donald Colbert, an MD, PhD and Midwesterner who'd spent most of his career at Cincinnati Children's Hospital as a virologist. Prior to Columbia, he served as chair of the department at the University of Texas Medical Center, Galveston, and had established an important federal biohazard facility that researched rare viral illnesses. He was a superior scientist and prolific author who'd written several textbooks, but importantly, he was not a native New Yorker, did not appreciate the ebb and flow of the job, or understand the complexities of life at Columbia. Honestly, very few do.

I liked Donald, and we developed an immediate rapport. One day, he asked if we could speak.

"Michael, I need your help. I want to remove London as head of transplant; I need to get rid of him. I have discussed the issue extensively with Dean Sterngold and Michael Winters, CEO of New York Presbyterian. They are concerned that if we fire him, he will engender litigation. We want you to consider stepping down as the head of oncology to become a vice chair of the department to work on important projects with me; I can certainly use your expertise in some many areas. This is not a demotion—you will remain an active leader in the division, and I'll increase your salary to show my gratitude."

"Can I think about it for a few days?"

"Of course, I have an office for you in the chairman's suite. We'll recruit a new division director, and I want you to take an active role in the recruitment process and selection of your successor.

Donald told me everyone expected London to leave rather than accept a demotion and salary reduction. "Give it some thought."

What choice did I have? None, really.

As I contemplated my future, I reasoned that I would retain my ability to see patients, the singular most important aspect of my work and my essence as a physician; I would continue my work with Hope & Heroes, also vitally important to me. I would, in my new role, be responsible for outreach and expanding the department's clinical operations, communications, and work with the Columbia University development people to increase philanthropy. I would yield control of the divisional operations and recognition as director, but I would no longer be responsible for all the crap and hospital mandatory bullshit. The positives seemed to outweigh the negatives; I told Donald, "I accept and look forward to working closely with you."

Colbert was thrilled.

London, as expected, resigned rather than accept demotion, and our strategy succeeded. He found another position at a second-rate Children's Hospital in the suburbs of New York City, a pedestrian institution. Good riddance.

Fred Le Ping, MD, PhD replaced me after my 15-year tenure as division director. He was a researcher from Harvard. His interests encompassed precision oncology with a focus on Columbia's Irving Cancer Center. His laboratory had identified cancer promoting genes and developed targeted therapy to knock out the abnormal gene pathways; his work was novel, innovative, and very cool. I asked Alan Goldman, Barry Hirsch, and Laura Hill, Boston friends and colleagues, about Le Ping, but no one knew him. He had no recent experience caring for patients and knew nothing about running a clinical service. He would not have been my choice. However, he had National Cancer Institute grant funding exceeding $5 million, an amount of money that bolstered the NIH ranking of the Irving Cancer Center and Department of Pediatrics significantly—an all-important measure. This fact alone made Le Ping an attractive candidate, regardless of all other parameters. He was offered the job.

First impressions: Le Ping was not committed to Columbia, had little respect for what I had accomplished, had no reverence for Hope & Heroes despite the fact the charity supported 40 percent of the divisional budget. He manhandled Cora Kenny, allowed the clinical enterprise to deteriorate, lost National Cancer Institute funding for his research, did not recruit a single clinician or scientist, poorly managed the divisional finances, and allowed the program to fall into a significant deficit. On the positive side, he did establish a first in class precision medicine program that identified abnormal and mutated tumor genes, and attempted to match new and existing chemotherapy and immunotherapy treatments to ameliorate the genetic abnormality. The program was cutting edge, ahead of its time, and exists today as Le Ping's legacy.

He lasted four years before accepting a position at Memorial Sloan Kettering as Chief of Pediatrics—go figure. However, prior to his departure, he decimated the division; eight Columbia faculty members resigned. Cora Kenny became the division director at Buffalo Children's, Roswell Park; Kim Levy, the head of the Survivor Wellness Program, went to Cornell; and six people went to Sloan Kettering, including Jacki Blade Gender and Nerissa Maria Angelo. I was crestfallen. Our once-extraordinary program slipped back into the abyss, and we spent two years in limbo.

The week prior to Le Ping's departure he had the audacity to attend a divisional pool party at Jacki Blade Gender's home in Scarsdale. He had just returned from Thailand and boasted that the purpose of his trip was to purchase suits because his new job at Sloan Kettering would be more corporate, formal, and he was expected to dress appropriately. In addition, he told his assembled prior colleagues and co-workers that Hope & Heroes was an afterthought, minor league compared to the fundraising efforts at Memorial.

"Have a nice life, Fred Le Ping."

Donald Colbert, feeling the stress of the world on his slender shoulders, decided to resign after a decade as chair; honestly, I have no clue as to how he lasted a full 10 years, but he did. The lack of hospital support and pressure from Dean Sterngold was intense; the department had a two to three million dollar deficit for three consecutive years, which was not acceptable. There was most definitely a trickle-down phenomenon that affected the entire department. One early morning I noticed Don in his office alone staring deeply into space, transfixed. The visual was reminiscent of a picture I recall of President John Kennedy, shoulders hunched, back to the photographer, alone in the Oval Office during the Cuban Missile Crisis. The fate of our nation and the entire world depended on his making the correct decision. Don undoubtedly concluded he needed change. He relinquished the chair to pursue his interest in global child safety and food insecurity, eventually becoming an associate dean at the Vagelos College of Medicine and director of the school's global health initiative. Perfect for him.

Evan Greene succeeded Colbert as chair of the department.

Evan is a New Yorker. Raised in Great Neck, Long Island, he attended Brown University for his MD and PhD, where he was a respectable intercollegiate swimmer. His graduate training was at Boston Children's and CHOP, though he came to Columbia via Texas Children's Hospital in Houston, where he was the Division Director of Allergy and Immunology. His research on "natural killer cells" and their important role in the body's innate defense against infection and cancers is groundbreaking. He was recently inducted into the prestigious National Academy of Science for his scientific contributions. When we first met, he told me that his first priority was to stabilize and rebuild pediatric oncology. I was an immediate convert.

Evan and I shared a sense of history; together we dedicated effort, time, and resources to restore our past and connect it to our future. The Babies Hospital, founded by twin sisters Sarah and Jacki McNutt in 1887, is the second oldest hospital dedicated to the care of children in the United States, and the first in New York. The list of discoveries and innovations is long and continues today as present faculty and researchers continue their pursuit of excellence inpatient care, education, and research. Evan and I believed it important to develop a sense of pride in Columbia Children's Health and the Department of Pediatrics, and the way forward was to recognize the past history of the former Babies Hospital.

This is the story we wanted to tell. But the challenge was great; in 1998, Columbia Presbyterian, including the Babies Hospital, merged with New York Hospital. The new entity, New York Presbyterian Hospital, brought together two Ivy League medical schools, Columbia University College of Physicians and Surgeons and Cornell University College of Medicine, and their affiliated hospitals. The singular goal was to establish and promote a monolithic brand, New York Presbyterian, without regard for the distinguished history encompassing more than 120 years.

Evan asked me to develop a marketing and branding initiative for the Department of Pediatrics. We created a philanthropic board, coined the name, Columbia Children's Health, and hired a public relations firm, Group Gordon, to serve as important members of the team. We developed a logo, tag line, started a community forum for referring pediatricians, increased social media communication, developed a monthly internal email newsletter called *The Check Up*, created divisional brochures for cardiology, gastroenterology, and hematology-oncology, and significantly increased philanthropy. Evan and I discussed writing the history of the Babies Hospital; I suggested that Beth Hanson, a marvelous writer and terrific colleague work on the project with me, and he agreed.

The story is not complete, much work remains to be done, and to this day we feel as if we are paddling upstream, underresourced and understaffed. But, we continue to pursue our dream and restore our department's bygone greatness.

My Turn

As a pediatric oncologist who specializes in leukemia and lymphoma, the most common cause for a new patient consultation is an enlarged lymph node in the neck. Thus, my experience has prepared me to make a fairly accurate assessment of a lymph node by recording its history and completing a physical examination. I recognize benign nodes and recommend observation or a course of antibiotics. I also recognize a lymph node of concern, and I know when to suggest an ultrasound, chest x-ray, a complete blood count, and a referral to one of the surgeons, Bob Johnson or Peter Karakos, for a biopsy. If I have learned anything in my 40 years of practice, it is the assessment of a child or adolescent with lymphadenopathy. I have an intuitive sense that distinguishes benign from malignant, reactive nodes, from lymphoma or Hodgkin's disease.

In February 2018, I felt a lymph node in my neck. It was just behind my right ear, about three centimeters in length and rubbery in texture. It was not tender, was not erythematous or painful. It was just inexplicably there. I wasn't sick; in fact, I felt extremely well. I did not have any evidence of an infection, no fever, no sweating and no weight loss. It was just there. I waited a few days, and then emailed my friend, the surgeon Hal Short, and told him I had a lymph node in an unusual location and asked if he would examine it for me. He emailed back and told me to come up to his office on the eighth floor of the Irving Pavilion at 2:30, when he would be finished in the operating room. I called his office, spoke to his assistant, Madeline, and told her that Dr. Short wanted to see me at 2:30. She asked me my medical record number and birthdate and told me to bring my insurance card. I asked, "Would you call my cell when Dr. Short is ready for me? My office is on the seventh floor, and I can be up to your office in a minute."

Madeline called me at 2:40. "Dr. Short is ready to see you now."

Hal led me into the procedure room. There was a surgical spotlight hanging from the ceiling, and glass cabinets filled with gauze, suture material, and the supplies that a surgeon would need for simple ambulatory procedures lined the walls. The examination table was in the center of the room.

We made small talk about kids and vacations. We had been friends for more than 20 years, had served on the same Columbia doctors university committees, and he had operated on me twice before for herniorrhaphies. He also performed the total thyroidectomy on my daughter, Lauren, during her own bout with cancer. I knew Hal well and trusted him. One of the things I liked best about him, aside from his extraordinary expertise as an endocrine surgeon with particular skill in performing the Whipple procedure for pancreatic cancer, was his calm demeanor.

"Let me see that lymph node that you're concerned about."

I sat on the exam table and turned my head to the left so he could see and feel the node in question.

"Well, I certainly feel what you are referring to. Is it tender? Is it bothering you at all?"

"What bothers me is that it is there, and I have no explanation for it. I feel perfectly fine. I just want to remove it."

"I really don't think it's anything to worry about. Let's wait a few weeks and see what happens to it."

"Hal, my intuition tells me that you should remove it now and do the biopsy; let's just do it. You know me. Just give me a little local lidocaine and take it out."

"Okay, take off your shirt and lie on the table with the right side of your neck up."

Dr. Short turned on the overhead surgical spotlight, took off his white coat, rolled up his sleeves, and took a sterile surgical equipment pack from the cabinet. He placed the pack unopened on a table and put on a pair of sterile gloves. A nurse entered the room and asked if he needed assistance, and he indicated that he could use a hand for a few minutes. The nurse placed a sterile drape on the table, opened a pack of 4 x 4 sterile gauze, poured betadine on the gauze, and held a vile of two percent lidocaine, so that he could withdraw the analgesic into a sterile syringe.

"Thanks, Lisette. I think I can manage from here," he said. "Before you go, though, please fill out a surgical pathology requisition form for Dr. Weiner and just place a jar of Bouin's solution with the top off on the table. I'll let you know when I'm done, and if you would, I want you to hand carry the sample to hemepath on VC-14."

"Just give me a call when you're done," Lisette said.

"Come back in about 10 minutes."

"Michael, are you okay?" he asked. "I'm going to get started."

I was cool, the procedure itself was a non-event. Years ago, I had several lipomas—benign fatty tumors—removed from my back with a spritz of local anesthetic; no big deal really. Regarding the anticipated result, it would be what it would be. Either way, it was beyond my control. If it is malignant, I figured that I'd rather know that day instead of three or four weeks from now. I was as relaxed as I could have been.

Hal cleaned my neck with the betadine, three times. He then positioned three sterile drapes on my neck, covering my face and hair and exposing the lymph node. He injected about 5 ml of lidocaine into and around the node for analgesia. He waited a few minutes for it to work and asked, "Do you feel this?"

"I feel nothing."

I felt Hal working diligently and deftly to make an incision, control the superficial bleeding, isolate and remove the node in one piece. He placed the tissue into the bottle containing the yellow colored Bouin's solution and showed it to me. "Here it is, a grayish-whitish lymph node."

This 2–3 cm piece of tissue in some odd way would dictate my future. Benign of malignant. I had nothing to do now, but wait.

I had not told Alicia that I had a lymph node on the back of my neck, behind my right ear, but now that we'd operated, there was no hiding it from her any longer. I had a small bandage at the biopsy sight. Typical of Alicia, she was not concerned, "You'll be fine, you're not sick. It's probably nothing to be worried about. Your father lived until he was 95 and your mother is 97. Don't think about it until you have to think about it."

"Easier said than done, but I'll try."

Ali Mahesh, the director of hematopathology at Columbia Presbyterian, is a really good guy. My relationship with him has always been excellent. We respect one another professionally and we are work friends. I have the utmost confidence in his ability to make an accurate diagnosis for the patients that I care for, so when he called me the day after the node biopsy I was a bit fearful, but ready to hear what he had to tell me.

Ali told me that he had reviewed the biopsy with Mehmet Erogan and Charles Anderson, and they both agreed the nodal tissue was consistent with a classical, low-grade follicular lymphoma. He indicated that he was going to do the special immunostains and flow on the node, but he wanted to call and give me the result personally. "The sample was put in Bouin's solution, but it should have been delivered on a gauze soaked in normal saline; we won't be able to do any sequencing or molecular testing. No harm done really, but you should mention it to Dr. Short. The final report will be in CROWN, the electronic medical record, by the end of the day."

Dr. Short's routine when extirpating a pancreas is to place the tissues for pathological diagnosis in Bouin's solution, not his fault, he merely did not know that lymph nodes should be processed in normal saline, and it did not occur to me to correct him; I was thinking of other things.

I anticipated a diagnosis of non-Hodgkin's lymphoma. My father, Bill, had a diffuse large cell B-cell lymphoma diagnosed at 92 years of age. He received six cycles of aggressive chemotherapy, lost his hair, but otherwise did incredibly well. He lived to die three years later from a subdural hematoma of his brain secondary to a fall. I expected to learn I had the same diagnosis. Thus, in an odd manner, I was relieved to hear the news. Fear, at least at this moment, was not an emotion I experienced.

"Thanks, Ali, for letting me know, I really appreciate it. I had a feeling this was not going to be benign; I was expecting some type of lymphoma."

"You should give Connor Williams or Craig Runkle a call."

"I will."

I knew both Drs. Williams and Runkle well. Connor was really smart, a wildcard, too arrogant for me, but he certainly knew non-Hodgkin's lymphoma inside and out. He was considered one of the foremost lymphoma specialists in the country and was the head of Columbia's lymphoma program. I have known Craig Runkle for almost 40 years. He is solid, sensible, experienced, and when my father was diagnosed with a diffuse large cell lymphoma 10 years ago, Craig was the first person I called. He also treated my cousin Richard Ross for Hodgkin's disease decades ago.

Connor was a bit too self-absorbed for my tastes. He traveled often, was frequently out of town, and I wasn't convinced that he would be adequately available. I would definitely speak to Craig, but I wasn't sure I wanted him as my doctor; we had too much history together. We were too close; it just did not feel right.

When Cathy Landers, Associate Director and Events Coordinator of Hope & Heroes, the charity I started more than 20 years ago, was diagnosed with Hodgkin's disease in November of 2017, I suggested Debra Lawrence. Debra worked with Connor Williams, was available, returned phone calls, and was quite knowledgeable. Working with Williams I thought she would discuss my case with Connor, thus I felt I was getting his expertise without his personality. I emailed Dr. Lawrence, explained that I had just been diagnosed with a follicular lymphoma and that I wanted to see her in consultation. She told me to call the office. I made an appointment for the next day.

I left my office early, knowing that Alicia would not be home. Tuesday afternoons she took our grandson, Wesley, to physical therapy. Clementine, our Cavalier King Charles Spaniel greeted me at the door. I grabbed her orange leash and took her for a walk along the Riverwalk in Hoboken. When we sold our house in Tenafly we found an apartment in the north end of Hoboken, a comfortable two-bedroom, nothing special. But the unobstructed views across the Hudson River of the Manhattan skyline, stretching from the George Washington Bridge to the Statue of Liberty, was arguably one of most spectacular panoramas anywhere in the world.

The day was chilly, but clear, and we walked for an hour. I needed to clear my head and get used to my new reality, I was now a cancer patient.

Alicia called my cell phone from her car at 5 p.m. and said she was on the way home. "Where are you?" she asked.

"Honey, just come home.

"Are you okay, did you get the result from the biopsy?"

"Just tired, please come home."

I heard Alicia put her key into the lock and I got up to greet her at the door. My facial expression could not hide the obvious. I told her I'd gotten the biopsy result and it was positive. I had a lymphoma.

My wife of almost 40 years, rather than sympathy, displayed an odd in-difference. Similar to my sister Margaret, Alicia refused to allow negative thoughts or energy into her space until she must. I am certain she was concerned; how could she not be?

"Are you alright? I mean really alright?"

I told her I was for the moment. The fact is I felt extraordinarily well, no symptoms, no fever, stable weight, no coughing. I was able to continue my full exercise routine. I was good.

I told her that I'd made an appointment to see an oncologist the next day, Debra Lawrence. "She's the doctor that took care of Cathy Landers; she seemed really good and attentive. I want you to go to the appointment with me, it's at 11."

She asked me if the lymphoma was the same as my father's. I told her no he had a diffuse large cell lymphoma.

"No, it's different; it's a follicular lymphoma, quite common, quite treatable."

"Mikey, I am certain you will be fine. You're so healthy, you're going to beat this. Just try to relax. What about dinner? We have to eat something, it's early. Let's go to Baumgartens in Edgewater."

Baumgartens is a special place for our family. The original restaurant is in Englewood the adjacent town to Tenafly, where Alicia and I raised our family after leaving the city and our apartment on 87th Street in 1992. It was originally an old-fashioned ice cream parlor that was bought by Steve Chan, a Chinese restauranteur who maintained the original ambi-ence, but added a fresh Asian menu. We really enjoyed the food and when Steve opened a second location in Edgewater, a short drive from Hoboken, we were thrilled. The Edgewater version attempts to emulate the old-fash-ioned ice cream parlor ambience with Formica-topped tables and a juke box in the corner.

It was early when we arrived, the restaurant was almost empty. We sat in a booth and the waiter placed menus on the table. We told him we didn't need the menus and were ready to order. "We'd like the duck crepe, vegetable roll, orange chicken, and the string beans with pork, one white rice and one brown rice."

Dinner, as always, was delicious; we needed comfort food tonight and nothing is as good and welcome as Baumgartens. For dessert we shared a hot fudge sundae. We talked little about my new diagnosis; frankly, we spoke hardly at all. Small talk about Lauren and Eli, we agreed not to discuss anything with the children, and absolutely not a word to my mother. One thing was absolutely apparent: my follicular lymphoma did not diminish my appetite. At least not tonight.

Alicia was correct in recalling the Weiner family's history of longevity. My grandfather Nathan lived into his 90s, as did his brother, Wolff. My father's sister, Rhoda, lived to 104 and my mother's mother, Doris, despite being a miserable person, lived to 92. Alicia's parents both died at much earlier ages. Her mother was in her mid 70s when she succumbed to complications of Parkinson's disease and her father Paul, a sadistic narcissist, died at 82, probably of heart failure. He had a very strong family history of early death, secondary to heart disease.

Calm, generally speaking, is not in my repertoire. However, I was able to keep it together and remain composed and tranquil.

Follicular lymphoma was an entity that I knew something about. Although unusual in children and adolescents I have diagnosed and treated several such patients. In one recent case in a teenage boy the disease was localized to a solitary node, removed by biopsy and managed by observation only and without additional therapy; the patient remains perfectly well and without recurrence to this day.

I began to read voraciously about follicular lymphoma. I read lay articles by writers at the Mayo Clinic, online articles submitted by the Leukemia and Lymphoma Society, *Up to Date*, an online resource and library of scientific papers, some of which were written by physician investigators that I knew personally. After several hours, my eyes were tired and my brain weary. Enough for tonight.

Dr. Lawrence's office was on the second floor of the Columbia Doctors' midtown offices at 51 West 51st Street. Columbia Doctors, the association of private physicians, and members of the full-time faculty, maintained offices in Midtown in order to be more convenient to patients who worked and lived on the Upper East or West Sides of Manhattan. Columbia Presbyterian, located in Washington Heights, was not convenient. The neighborhood, mostly Dominican and indigent, had a reputation as being unsafe; therefore, to attract insured patients ambulatory offices and an outpatient surgery center were opened downtown. The model worked; private patients were pleased, as were the physicians and hospital.

We arrived a few minutes early, I registered, completed the obligatory forms, handed the receptionist my insurance card, and waited. One of the nurses came to the waiting area, called my name, and asked me to follow her to an exam room. She introduced herself, "My name is Barbara, I'm going to take your vital signs. Take your shoes off and get on the scale."

Weight, 200 lbs.; BP, 135/80; pulse, 68; temperature, 98.6.

"The doctor will be with you in a few minutes."

Dr. Debra Lawrence entered the exam room and introduced herself to Alicia and me. She sat down in the chair at the desk in front of the computer screen, I sat next to the desk, and Alicia sat in the corner. My first impression, "My goodness you are so young."

She was a small, dark-haired young woman, smartly dressed and very personable. I liked her immediately. I retold the history of the present illness, and she told me that she had reviewed my medical history and medications in preparation for the consultation. This information is available on CROWN, the hospital's electronic, computerized medical record. She also said that she'd spoken with Dr. Mahesh to confirm the diagnosis and, in fact, had personally reviewed the pathology slides with him. I was impressed.

"I want to examine you," she said. "Take off your shirt. Do you need a gown?"

"No, not really," I replied, and got onto the exam table.

The doctor looked in my ears with the otoscope, and in my mouth. She palpated my neck, noted the scar behind my right ear, and told me that she believed there was a second node in the submental region underneath my chin. It was very small and she said she was unsure of its significance. She listened to my heart and lungs, and then palpated my abdomen.

Dr. Lawrence told me there was little doubt that I had a follicular lymphoma.

"You need to have some tests for staging purposes," she said. "PET/CT and I would probably do a bone marrow aspirate and biopsy. You will also need some additional blood work: CBC, LFT's, chemical profile, LDH, Beta 2 microglobulin, ESR, and CRP. I can have my nurse draw the bloods now and if you are ready I can do the bone marrows now as well, up to you."

I told her I needed a little time to process. "I'll get the bloods drawn tomorrow morning from one of my nurses and I'd like to postpone the marrow for a day or so if possible," I said. I asked if I could have the PET/CT and the bone marrow at the hospital uptown.

"No worries, I need to make the arrangements to accommodate you. I need to make a few calls."

Dr. Lawrence told me she believed that I had localized, low-grade follicular lymphoma. It is not a curable illness, but one can expect long periods of disease remission, relapses and re-treatment. Some believe that low stage disease observation without treatment is acceptable management until you become symptomatic or demonstrate advancing symptoms. She suggested that we meet again when we had all the results to make some decisions. "I would be optimistic that you will be okay," she said. "Here is my mobile cell number, call me or message me anytime. Let me have your number as well."

"May I call you Debra?"

"Of course."

Alicia and I stood to leave. I told Debra that I could not consider observation only; medically and psychologically I would not be able to rest if I did not receive therapy with cure as the objective.

We stopped at the front desk. The receptionist told me she would schedule the tests and apologized for asking me to collect the $30 co-pay for the visit.

"No worries." I handed the receptionist my American Express card.

We left the office and walked across the street to the Sea Grill at Rockefeller Center for lunch. I had my usual Virgin Mary; Alicia had a Bloody Mary with Tito's vodka. I had fish and chips; Alicia ordered mussels.

We talked about the visit with the doctor and how we had heard different things. I had heard that follicular lymphoma was not curable, while Alicia had heard that I would be fine. Isn't it interesting that two people hearing the same thing from the doctor interpret things differently? People hear what they want to hear and their psycho-emotional constitution influences the message.

Now What?

Where to begin? Who to trust? What questions to ask? Where to turn for answers? The experience of actually having cancer was different from anything I had previously endured. It was certainly different than treating my own cancer patients; different than my experience guiding Lauren through her own cancer decision-making process; different from being by my father's side when he was diagnosed with lymphoma. This time it was me—I was the patient. The diagnosis represented a threat to my life, my time with Alicia, Lauren, Eli, and grandchildren. This time, I was not the one with the answers.

I needed to stay busy. My patients, meetings, phone calls, and work provided some distraction as I tried to keep my mind on anything except my cancer. Still, it was hard to do. I made lists of things to do, people to speak to, doctors to consult. I knew with certainty that I would receive my treatment at Columbia; there was no question about that. Columbia University Irving Medical Center had been my home for decades, and I would be able to expedite appointments, tests, and procedures, allowing me some modicum of control—a valuable commodity.

Debra Lawrence appreciated my need to consult with others and agreed that we would make therapeutic decisions together when my due diligence was complete; Craig Runkle was on the top of my list, as was Cary Frost.

Craig was sensible and had good judgment—not necessarily a harbinger of academic minutia, just a really solid clinician, the type upon which Columbia Presbyterian's reputation for excellence was grounded. His expertise was lymphoma. When my father Bill was diagnosed with a diffuse large cell lymphoma, Craig was his doctor. I trusted him.

I walked up the back stairs to Dr. Runkle's office on the ninth floor of Irving Pavilion. His office door was open, and he was sitting behind his desk, waiting for me. He was tall—6 foot, 3—with straight gray hair and dark glasses, predictably dressed in a blue shirt, a tie, and a white coat. His office was comfortable; not large, but pleasant, bathed in a soft warm light from the green-glass banker's lamp on his desk.

I told Craig before our appointment that I had been diagnosed with a follicular lymphoma. He had my electronic chart open on the screen and agreed that I needed a PET/CT scan, a bone marrow aspirate, and a biopsy. I told him that I had seen Debra Lawrence and wanted her to be my doctor, and he agreed that it was a good idea, telling me that although she was young, she was also capable, likeable, and had a calm approach with patients. We talked about therapeutic options, observation, Rituximab, radiotherapy, and chemotherapy, and decided to speak again when the remaining test results were available.

"Thanks, Craig. I appreciate it," I said, shaking his hand and turning to leave.

"Of course. You'll be fine," he encouraged. "Relax."

I stopped at his assistant's desk across the hall with my American Express in hand for the $30 co-pay. She told me that Dr. Runkle was not charging me for the visit.

In my career I have performed thousands of bone marrow aspirates and biopsies, and that is a conservative estimate. When I was a fellow at Johns Hopkins in 1976, my research project necessitated normal bone marrow stem cells. My mentor, Lyle Sensenbrenner, performed the procedure on me to retrieve cells for culture, which we then placed in a chamber and embedded in the abdominal cavity of mice for an optimal growth environment. The procedure is straightforward and takes just few minutes. However, it is not without discomfort. The aspirate uses a large-bore needle with a sharp cutting edge to penetrate the bone cortex and enter the central medullary cavity, the soft, liquid cellular proliferative compartment where our blood cells are manufactured. The biopsy uses a Jamshidi needle to remove a solid core of bone marrow to be analyzed by hematopathologists.

Dr. Lawrence scheduled my test for Monday morning in the Irving Pavilion Garden.

"Good morning. You ready?"

"Yup, let's do this."

The nondescript exam treatment room was similar to so many others—a desk with a computer, an exam table, a wall-mounted otoscope, and an ophthalmoscope. I removed my pants and climbed onto the table on my right side. Debra asked if I had any questions.

"Nope."

After placing a sterile drape, she cleaned the area, the left posterior iliac crest, with betadine.

"I'm gonna use two percent lidocaine. Ready for a prick?"

I closed my eyes, took deep breaths to relax, and recited my mantra, "SHER-ING," a nonsense word I had learned years ago when I practiced transcendental meditation.

"I'm gonna begin and do the aspirate first."

I felt nothing, nada, zilch. The biopsy, similarly, was quick, easy, and painless.

"Great job, Debra!" I was relieved.

The PET/CT was scheduled for the next morning. The scanner was located in the sub-basement of the of the Allan Rosenfield Building of the Columbia University's School of Public Health; the location is not convenient to anything.

A positron emission tomography, or PET scan, is an imaging test that uses a radioactive drug tracer tagged to a glucose moiety, as tumor cells consume more sugar than healthy cells. When the radiotracer is broken down, positrons are emitted and gamma rays produced. The PET scanner can pick up the emitted gamma rays and merge images with the CT to compose an accurate image map of the internal orans and structures.

I arrived early, completed the obligatory demographic and insurance paperwork, and followed the technician into a quiet prep room. An IV was inserted into my left forearm, the radiotracer administered, and I was instructed to drink the gastrografin over the next 60 minutes. Once in the scanner, the entire test was completed in less than a half hour.

That afternoon, Debra called my cell phone. "Good news," she said. "The bone marrow is negative, there's no evidence of lymphoma. The PET/CT is positive in your neck only, actually two distinct nodes, but no evidence of disease in any other anatomic site. Why don't you come to the office tomorrow and we can review some options for treatment?"

Smiling broadly, I sighed with relief and relaxed for the first time since Hal Short had done the biopsy in his treatment room. "Thanks, Debra. I'll see you tomorrow."

Low stage, absence of symptoms, no adverse serum markers, negative cytogenetics, and no abnormal molecular findings. For the first time since diagnosis, I believed I would be a survivor, a long-term survivor.

But, I reminded myself, *there is no cure.*

Alicia accompanied me to the appointment the next morning. Debra reiterated that I had Stage 2, favorable follicular lymphoma; observation-only was not an option and, at this time, chemotherapy was similarly off the table. She suggested I speak with Mark David, the radiotherapist who managed the lymphoma cases, and get his opinion. Another option was Rituximab, an anti-CD 20 monoclonal antibody administered weekly for four doses, then every month for one year. Debra again indicated that, historically, follicular lymphoma was incurable but generally ran a chronic course of remission, exacerbation, re-treatment, and remission, followed by another recurrence. In addition, she told us that there was also about a 25 percent conversion to diffuse large cell non-Hodgkin's lymphoma.

That information was unsettling.

Diffuse large cell NHL is an acute lymphoma that I preferred not to have to deal with—not now or ever. It necessitated six to eight months of aggressive, multi-agent chemotherapy, and although cure rates approached 70 percent, there was definite mortality. The side effects of treatment were real and not insignificant. Immediate toxicities included nausea and vomiting, total alopecia, pancytopenia, mucositis, and risk of overwhelming infections; whereas the long-term complications were liver and heart damage and the risk of secondary, treatment-related malignancies. As an oncologist this was not information I did not already know, unsettling to say the least.

Welcome to the world of the cancer patient: too many options to contemplate, no guarantees, indecision at every turn, a changing landscape, a dizzying experience. How does one decide the path forward, the path to a cure? I told Debra that I would make an appointment with Mark David and that I wanted to see Cary Frost as well. She agreed.

I decided to begin a diary. I recorded facts, questions, thoughts, discussions, etc. I also decided to develop a personal cancer lexicon. *Indecision* was the first word on my list.

As Alicia and I left the office, my wife, confidant, and best friend of 40 years repeated, "You will be fine."

All I heard was, *no cure.*

I called Dr. David's office and the receptionist told me that the doctor had been expecting my call and asked if I was available to come in that afternoon.

"Yes, tell me the time."

"Does 2 p.m. work? Do you know where we are located?"

"Yes. See you at 2."

David was waiting for me. I followed him into his office in the basement of the Children's Hospital North Building. Mark David is a colleague with whom I share patients; his expertise, similar to mine, is non-Hodgkin's lymphoma and Hodgkin's disease. His office, windowless and without ambient light, was noticeably bright, with three lamps and a large ceiling-mounted fluorescent beaming. He told me he had reviewed my PET/CT scan and believed that he could effectively treat both nodal areas in my neck in one field. He was confident that localized follicular lymphoma radiation as a single modality offered a cure rate that approached 80 percent. He had my attention. Cure was my goal.

We walked across the hallway to an exam room that was dark and nondescript. The nurse took my vital signs and David examined my neck.

"No problem, this will be straightforward," he said.

I asked a number of rapid-fire questions. "What dosage? How many sessions? Will my thyroid be in the field?"

"Relax, slow down," he answered.

I trusted David to treat my teenage and young patients, but did I trust him to treat me? I was terrified of radiotherapy. It has a place in the armamentarium of cancer therapy modalities, but the toxicities, immediate and long-term, are real. RT gave me pause.

David told me his plan was to give 2,100 centigray—the measure of energy—1 field, 10 sessions in a 2-week period. The thyroid, out of necessity, would be in the field. Expected side effects were fatigue, hair loss in the field, possible mucositis, and a sore throat.

I could deal with lethargy, fatigue, mouth sores, and the worst sore throat imaginable; these side effects were a small price to pay for cure. But the risk of second cancers and vascular disease was not insignificant and frightened me. I have cared for several patients with Hodgkin's disease who received involved field low-dose RT to the neck and developed thyroid cancer. Similarly, it has been established that survivors of Hiroshima and Nagasaki, or of nuclear reactor accidents like Chernobyl and Fukushima, have a seven-fold increase risk of thyroid cancer. The medical literature is replete with studies confirming that low to moderate doses of irradiation increases the risk of papillary thyroid cancer significantly. Radiotherapy causes vascular narrowing, induces intimal wall inflammation and predisposes patients to cardiovascular disease and stroke.

"David, I need time to think."

Leaving the Department of Radiotherapy, I saw no obvious pathway. Was it worthwhile to risk another potential bout of cancer—and this time worse than anything I was currently dealing with—for the possibility of a total cure? There was no certainty; indecision prevailed.

Cary Frost, chief of the lymphoma service at Cornell, is undoubtedly one of the foremost experts in the city, with a reputation that is internationally renowned. I valued his opinion. We spoke on the phone, and he asked to review my records prior to my visit. I scanned and emailed him the pathology, molecular genetics, blood, bone marrow, and PET/CT scan results.

In 1998, New York Hospital, Weill Cornell and Columbia Presbyterian, and Columbia University College of Physicians and Surgeons merged to form the New York Presbyterian Hospital. The two associated Ivy League medical schools remained separate and independent. The foundation of the merger was financial. Both institutions had been flirting with mounting operating losses, bad publicity, poor public perception, and pending litigations. In the world of hospitals, bigger is better—economy of scale and enhanced bargaining power with insurers and vendors would ensure the long-term viability of both institutions. The merger made sense, however, the hoped-for integration of clinical services has never actually been realized.

On the ground, in the trenches, the institutions are competitors, a division made more obvious by their starkly different cultures. Compared to Columbia, Cornell seemed rigid and old school. Their faculty wore three-piece suits and watch fobs and ate their lunch in a wood-paneled doctors' dining room with white tablecloths and waiter service. Columbia, on the other hand, was less formal and more diverse. Most of the staff wore open-collar shirts and white coats; a physicians' dining room did not exist and most doctors ate at their desks if they took the time for lunch at all. Despite these internal disparities, the merged entity flourished. New York Presbyterian is a corporate financial juggernaut, ranked among the top five hospitals in the country by *U.S. News & World Report*.

Cary's office was on the third floor of the Starr Building, the ambulatory edifice for Weill Cornell faculty practice physicians. As I stepped off the elevator, registered as a new patient, and sat in the waiting room, I was struck by the sameness of the patients and staff. They were almost all white. Cornell, located on York Avenue in the 70s, provided care to the carriage trade of the Upper East Side of Manhattan: wealthy Caucasians. Columbia served the Latino communities of Washington Heights and the south Bronx, as well as a diverse Muslim and Asian immigrant population; the faces were black, brown, yellow, and white.

"Michael, come on in."

Dr. Frost reviewed my records and told me that he agreed with the diagnosis of early stage favorable follicular lymphoma.

"Michael, I like to tell my patients that they will not die from follicular lymphoma; they will die *with* follicular lymphoma."

It was difficult to gain control of my emotions. This was not unexpected, but that did not make it easier. I was confused, frightened, and afraid of what would be my future. There was certainty—no doubt I had cancer; another word to the lexicon: *acceptance*.

He reiterated identical therapeutic options: initial observation until symptomatic, Rituximab, radiation therapy, single agent Bendamustine chemotherapy.

"Cary, I want to be a patient, not a doctor. Tell me, what would you do? You make the decision, but observation is off the table; there's no way I could do nothing."

"Well, you don't need chemotherapy. For your stage and disease characteristics, irradiation could be curative, but I am not an advocate of RT alone. You know follicular lymphoma is a systematic disease and despite the absence of symptoms and other anatomic sites, I favor Rituximab alone or in combination with RT. I'd like you to speak with Dr. Lloyd at Memorial Sloan Kettering. I'll make the introduction and share your records with him."

I contacted Lloyd's office and asked his assistant if we could arrange a conference call. Frankly, I did not see the need to see him in person, my history is non-contributory and there was nothing of note to be gained by another physical exam. I needed his opinion after a review of the records. Lloyd agreed. We scheduled a call for the next morning, and I asked Debra Lawrence to join and she willingly agreed.

After our introductions, Lloyd told me and Debra that he had reviewed the materials and spoken with Cary Frost. They concurred that Rituximab weekly times four dosages and low-dose involved field irradiation was the best course of action. Debra and I felt comfortable. I agreed. I would submit to the RT. I called Craig Runkle to inform him of our decision, and he agreed as well. Treatment was scheduled to begin the following Monday.

The next word in my lexicon: *trust*. I trusted the collective decision of my doctors. Still, I was determined not to die with follicular lymphoma; my single-minded focus was cure.

I arrived at the oncology infusion center on the 14th floor of the Irving Pavilion at 8 a.m., accompanied by Alicia. The center was on the top floor of the building; the unit had been the executive suite of Columbia Presbyterian. The offices had been large with spectacular, unobstructed views of the New York City skyline to the south, and directly to the west, the George Washington Bridge to New Jersey rose above the Hudson River. I stopped at the registration desk to check in. They seemed to be expecting me.

The waiting room was jam-packed with patients, escorts, and companions; people of all different sizes, shapes, and colors. It was one of the things I loved about Columbia, I thought, sitting in quiet observation. My patients in pediatric oncology were multiracial, multicultural, and multilingual, but as patients, we were all the same. How different it was from Cornell.

Every chair in the waiting room was occupied, but no one spoke. The three wall-mounted TVs were each tuned to a different channel—CNN, *The Today Show* on NBC, and *Good Morning America* on ABC—but they were little more than white noise as no one was watching.

Before long, a smiling woman approached. Extending her hand, she introduced herself. "I'm Josie. You must be Dr. Weiner, Mrs. Weiner. Come with me to area H. I'm all set up for your treatment."

Area H was one of 12 treatment sections. Each section had six reclining lounges with a small TV affixed to a movable, collapsible arm, a locker for personal belongings, and a privacy curtain. Alicia sat in an adjacent chair as Josie started an IV in my left forearm, successful on her first attempt.

"Dr. Lawrence ordered Benadryl orally and dexamethasone IV as premeds and I assume you know the first Rituximab infusion is given slowly over six hours."

Rituximab belongs to a class of drugs called monoclonal antibodies. Tumor cells, specifically B-cell lymphoma cells, have a receptor or protein, CD20, on their surface. Rituximab is a man-made antibody developed using recombinant DNA technology. It attaches to the CD20 receptor and causes the tumor cells to disintegrate, inhibiting the production of new tumor cells. Side effects include allergic reactions, nausea, muscle aches and pain, and predisposition to infections, thus the Benadryl and steroids.

I positioned the recliner for maximum comfort, Alicia wrapped me in two blankets and placed a pillow under my head; I quickly fell asleep. I woke intermittently while Alicia meandered, wandering over to my office on the seventh floor to use my computer and bringing me a yogurt for lunch. At 3 p.m., I was finished; tired, but done for the day. It had been easy with no untoward effects. We drove home together, Alicia behind the wheel.

I tolerated the four infusions of Rituximab without issue or side effects. But I realized that although the infusion center was overflowing with humanity, patients were alone—alone with their thoughts, alone with their fear, alone with chemotherapy and needles, and alone with the nausea. I too felt alone and added another word to my list: *isolation*. Cancer patients navigate their experience alone. Family, friends, and colleagues may be present to offer support, but the experience is yours alone. They can hold your hand, offer encouragement, wipe up the vomit, and bring lunch, but I realized that it's just me.

The irradiation was scheduled to begin three to four weeks hence. I possessed a single-minded determination to not allow negative thoughts into my psyche. I accepted my cancer diagnosis and was determined to allow my body and mind to acknowledge the cancer and work to mitigate its effects. I remained undeterred in my quest for cure.

The concept of fighting cancer or battling the disease for me did not work. Remaining calm and tranquil and keeping my routine as normal as possible was my path forward. I adopted a proactive approach, embracing complementary medical practices to augment and enhance the traditional treatments of immunotherapy and irradiation. I meditated daily, had thrice weekly acupuncture, altered my diet to primarily, but not rigidly, vegetarian and to include foods high in antioxidants and low in animal fats. I added the anti-inflammatory supplement turmeric and vitamin D to augment the positive effects of Rituximab. I am a strong advocate of integrative therapies and have been for 20 years, since Cora Kenny and I began the first integrative therapies program in the country for patients with cancer and their families. The clinic remains to this day the benchmark program in the United States and, under the leadership of Elana Ladas, has expanded to more than a dozen countries worldwide.

The Herbert Irving Cancer Center radiotherapy treatment facility is in the sub-basement. The designated elevator is located adjacent to the hospital's non-denominational chapel; I pressed SB. I arrived early for my simulation appointment, stopped at the reception desk, and my paperwork was in order. I signed the obligatory endless documents and the registrar made a copy of my insurance card. I sat in the comfortable, newly renovated waiting area and bathed in sunshine from the skylight.

My nurse, Carmen, an affable, petite Latina, handed me the consent form, already completed, minus my signature. I reluctantly signed. I continued to have trepidation, not regarding the immediate side effects, but the delayed, long-term toxicity.

"We'll do the simulation today," Carmen said. "It takes about an hour and a half, and then we'll need a few days to complete the calculations. Let's begin treatments Monday morning, with 10 daily sessions. We open at 7 a.m. I recommend you take that time, there's never a wait and you'll be less likely to see anyone you know."

Simulation is the process by which the radiation treatment fields are defined, filmed, and marked. The simulator is a large-bore computed tomography (CT) scanner that is used to contour the area to be treated. The physicist reviews the images, customizes the radiation beams, and individualizes the treatment for each unique patient. Positioning is extremely important.

"To stabilize your position we're gonna use a special immobilization device on the treatment table," Carmen said. She explained that I needed a custom-made, thermoplastic mask, precisely fit to my face to secure me to the table and hold my head in the correct position to ensure the accurate delivery of the radiation beam.

I removed my shirt. Carmen and Andy, an RT tech, helped me lie down on the treatment table. It, along with the room itself, was intolerably cold, like an ice bath or a meat refrigerator, designed to keep the equipment from overheating. I jumped up, Carmen and Andy laughed knowingly.

"We can put a blanket on the table under your back and another to cover you, but your neck and head must be flat, no sheets or blanket—try your best."

I got back on the table, more comfortable with the blankets, but still cold. Andy, a handsome, middle-aged African-American man, wore dark blue scrubs and a white coat with his name in script under the New York Presbyterian logo; he positioned me correctly. He placed a warm, wet plastic mesh film over my head, face, and neck. The mesh had openings for my eyes and nose, so I was able to see and breathe normally while being fitted. I lay motionless, and after about 15 minutes, the warm, soft, pliable radiation mask cooled and hardened. Andy bolted my mask to the table to assure immobility, and the Varian beam scanner moved in an arc overhead, from side to side, taking serial images and sending them to the computer for analysis and calculations. The process called dosimetry defines the treatment fields to maximize the dose of radiation to the area of the lymphoma and minimize the dose to the normal surrounding tissues.

The Varian beam whirred from side to side—noisy, but tolerable. My eyes, and only my eyes, followed the beam, and I almost expected to see magic bullets emitted from the large gray machine; bullets that would eradicate my cancer, I hoped. Failing to see mystical rays, I wondered and silently prayed that the irradiation was working. I attempted to meditate, repeated my mantra, concentrated on my breathing, and let my mind wonder. I was again alone, isolated. The motion of the Varian beam stopped and Carmen and Andy unbolted the mask. I was still freezing but elated. One down, nine treatments to go.

"See you tomorrow."

————————

The first week went easily, I arrived early, repeated the routine, and was in my office by 7:30, ready to resume a normal day. Then it hit me—the worst sore throat imaginable, no saliva, unable to swallow, barely able to speak. Lozenges, gargles, nothing worked. There was no relief; but there was also no other option. Treatment had to continue unabated and without hiatus. Alone, I meditated, followed the beam, looking for the magical killing rays—not there, but my throat belied their absence.

The second week of treatment ended as unceremoniously as it began, with me, cold and alone. The radiation-induced sore throat gradually improved, but as it did, I began to experience extreme lethargy. I was not tired in the way one might feel after a poor night's sleep, but was exhausted, dragging. My routine now disrupted, I had no choice but to rest and sleep. I tried to work, but was unable to do so, and frankly, it was unwise and dangerous to drive. Radiotherapy-induced fatigue is a strange if not uncommon phenomenon in patients. It is little understood and its etiology, mechanisms, and risk factors remain elusive, with this symptom in particular, poorly managed. The only known treatment is rest and time. I was patient. The extreme lethargy lasted three weeks then gradually abated.

Dr. Lawrence sent an email asking me to make an appointment for post-treatment evaluation four weeks hence. She scheduled a PET/CT and ordered a battery of blood work to assess response. The scan was scheduled for 9 a.m. Prior to the visit at 1 p.m., I felt well and healthy; I had regained my appetite, started to exercise, and returned to full-time work, seeing patients and fulfilling all responsibilities. But I was still a cancer patient and the thought of follow-up blood work and scans terrified me.

As a cancer doctor, I knew that certain tests, scans, and exams frightened every cancer patient—the Sword of Damocles syndrome, so named from Greek mythology. The fable recounts the story of Damocles, surrounded by joy and mirth, when Dionysus suspends a sword over his neck and head. Preoccupied with the danger of the sword, Damocles is unable to enjoy the beauty around him. This profound outlook is shared by survivors of childhood and adult cancers; and now it was shared by me.

Thankfully, my tests went well. Dr. Lawrence told me that the blood work and every test was normal or negative. The PET/CT similarly demonstrated no evidence of follicular lymphoma. But she told me there was a new finding: a nodule in my thyroid gland not present prior to radiotherapy. I knew it, just knew it—irradiation-induced thyroid cancer. I was not prepared for this, the saga continued.

Now what?

I made an appointment with Tom James, Lauren's doctor. He examined me, repeated the thyroid ultrasound in his office and confirmed the presence of a 6 millimeter solitary nodule. He told me that there was nothing to do at this time, the nodule was too small for biopsy and it was difficult to know for certain what the nodule represented. He indicated that about a third of such nodules are papillary thyroid carcinoma, the remainder benign cysts.

"What do we do?"

"Nothing, we observe, wait."

Acceptance, patience, isolation, the saga continues.

ARIELLA COLON

Mother And Daughter

"Who has Ariella Colon today?"

"I do," said Katie Green, pushing the video translator.

"Who is her floor nurse?" Lisa Jones asked, moving the portable computer cow and plugging it into a wall socket outside the room.

Sandra, her assigned nurse, joined rounds. "I am," she said. "Ariella had a good night, has remained afebrile with stable vital signs, and is asking to go home, which seems like a good indication that she is feeling well."

"What is her white count and absolute neutrophil count today?" I asked "Are her cultures negative?"

"Yes, the counts have recovered. She hasn't had a fever for over 48 hours, and the blood cultures are all negative," Katie replied.

"Lisa, when do they need to come back to clinic?"

"Tuesday to see Danica."

We entered Room 502. It was spotless. Mrs. Colon took great care in keeping Ariella's room clean. The hospital provides environmental services to clean each room each day, but the facilities people do a cursory job, mopping the floor, and cleaning the bathroom. It's up to the parents and family to keep their child's room clean. Some patient rooms are so filthy that it's appalling—old, dried food on the counters and desk, toys, books, and clothes strewn everywhere, the parent pullout bed unmade for days at a time. This was not the case with Ariella Colon's room. Everything was in its place, and despite the fact that this admission was a short two-day stay, the walls were decorated with personal cards, family pictures, and Ariella's artwork.

I greeted Ariella and Mrs. Colon. *"Buenos dias. ¿Como estas? ¿Queire ir a tu casa hoy?"*

Mrs. Colon smiled and clearly understood my few words of Spanish. I have a long and undistinguished history with the Spanish language. I began my Spanish studies in the seventh grade at the Grand Avenue Middle School before continuing on at W.C. Mepham High School in Merrick, Long Island. I was a horrible Spanish student. At Dickinson, I took a Spanish placement test, and despite five years of previous study, I placed in an introductory class and was forced to take four semesters of college Spanish in order to graduate. The only C's I received in college were in Spanish.

Charlie connected the video translator that allowed us to speak in real time to Ariella and her mother. We repeated to the Pacific interpreter that Ariella was discharged and should return to clinic next Tuesday.

Mrs. Colon understood. *"Gracias."*

Ariella's case had been unusual since day one. Her peripheral blood flow and initial complete blood count were consistent with acute lymphoblastic leukemia of B-cell lineage, but the confirmatory bone marrow aspirate and biopsy was inadequate and virtually acellular. I have successfully performed thousands of these procedures throughout my career—most flawlessly, but occasionally at the time of the diagnostic marrow, with difficulty—and I was always successful in obtaining sufficient material to make the diagnosis.

Ariella was different. The aspirated marrow from her iliac crest yielded a paucity of cells, barely sufficient to make slides and determine an accurate immunophenotype. The biopsy, despite more pressure and strength than I possessed, was similarly incredibly difficult to perform and the marrow core was fragmented. The hematopathologists at Columbia are excellent, slow and deliberate, but accurate. Drs. Mahesh and Anderson were able to confirm standard risk B-cell ALL, but were confounded by the high degree of necrosis, indicative of dying cells. We sent a bone marrow sample to the Dana-Farber Cancer Institute for their scientists to develop an individual leukemia cell profile for subsequent MRD (minimal residual disease), a reliable indicator of risk, complete remission, and potential for cure. Although they were unable to develop a personal cell-line profile, we decided to begin treatment in accordance with protocol.

We joined the DFCI consortium, started about 25 years ago by Alan Goldman, rather than enroll our cases onto the COG, Children's Oncology Group, protocols. The reason was two-fold. First, Alan is a personal friend and we favor the protocol for its straightforward approach and excellent results. Second, I thought there would be greater opportunity for career advancement for Cora Kenny and the young attendings in our division. The decision proved to be correct; Cora represented the interests of Columbia, and was recognized as a valued colleague and clinical investigator. But most importantly, the cure rates for children enrolled into these clinical trials are among the best results reported.

Although Ariella's case was atypical, she was eligible for the DFCI protocol. I can clearly recall introducing the idea to Mrs. Colon; it remains clearly engrained in my memory. Dr. Danica Boyko, an extraordinary first-year fellow, Lisa Jones, Susan Garfield, the first-year resident, and I met with Señora Colon in the meditation room on Tower 5. Her father, Señor Colon, was in the Dominican Republic and participated in the discussion via speakerphone. Danica and Susan, both fluent in Spanish, made the discussion less awkward and more personal. We discussed test results, an overview of the treatment, its expected results, and potential side effects.

The meditation room sits adjacent to the elevators in the lobby on the fifth floor. It is small, has no windows, and is crammed full with three comfortable armchairs and a small, two-person sofa. It may not be comfortably spacious, but it is the only room on the floor that ensures privacy during more serious conversations. There is a larger all-purpose space on the fifth floor, which is much more comfortable with windows that overlook the garden, but it also serves as a community space with a refrigerator, microwave, vending machine, bathroom, TV, and four tables and chairs. In addition to parents and visitors using the appliances and the communal restroom constantly, it is also a favorite spot for New York Presbyterian Hospital transporters and environmental service workers to relax and sleep in the comfortable chairs. Thus, while it may be more comfortable, it lacks the privacy necessary for conversations like the one we needed to have.

Mrs. Colon did not understand or speak English very well and preferred to speak Spanish. New York Presbyterian and Columbia University Medical Center have rules and regulations about disseminating information to non-English speaking patients and families, and they provide a mobile phone voice-interpreter service, as well as a video service, to assist the physicians and staff in their conduct of important discussions. Despite the best and most honest intentions of the interpreters, I remained skeptical that my words were translated as precisely and accurately as I might have liked. Perhaps it was my paranoia, but most assuredly, the interpretation generally lacked necessary compassion and emotion. Fortunately, the linguistic acumen of Danica and Susan mitigated my concerns—the conversation went as well as one might expect, all things considered.

"Mrs. Colon, Ariella has leukemia," I had told her. "Leukemia is a cancer of the bone marrow, or blood factory, and the kind of leukemia that Ariella has is called acute lymphoblastic leukemia. We refer to this type of leukemia as ALL. It is the most common type of leukemia in children and also the most treatable and curable." I paused to allow Susan to translate. Mrs. Colon, a pharmacist with medical knowledge, did not seem surprised.

She had suspected that her daughter might have leukemia and seemed relieved to learn it was ALL and not acute myelogenous leukemia, a less common and more difficult-to-treat type of leukemia in children with a significantly poorer rate of survival.

"The cause of ALL is not known. We do know that it is not secondary to anything you did or did not do as a parent. As far as we know, it is not caused by any environmental exposure and is not hereditary. It is possible that there may be a gene mutation, but that is hypothetical. Your other children are not at any increased risk of developing leukemia, so please don't be concerned about them." I allowed Susan to interpret my comments and ask if Mrs. Colon had any questions at this point.

"No hay preguntas."

I continued, "We would like to enroll Ariella in a clinical trial through the Dana-Farber Cancer Institute. The results of treatment are excellent, and we expect Ariella to tolerate the therapy and to have a cure rate of 90 percent. Ariella has standard risk characteristics—10 years old, initial white blood cell count of less than 50,000, B-lineage, and negative cerebrospinal fluid; all parameters are excellent prognostic variables."

I explained that treatment is divided into five phases: induction, consolidation I, central nervous system prophylaxis, consolidation II, and continuation. I wrote some notes in English, outlining what I had said. I have found that parents are not able to remain focused on the conversation once they learn that their child has leukemia, or any type of cancer for that matter, and if they are able to refer to the notes later on, they find it very helpful. Danica said that she would translate the notes for Mrs. Colon when we were finished.

Lisa Jones handed Mrs. Colon the DFCI protocol outline and consent form in Spanish. Lisa told her that we needed the signed consent form before enrolling Ariella in the study, to send samples of Ariella's bone marrow to Boston for analysis, and for the Columbia tumor bank for future research and molecular genetic testing. Danica, in Spanish, added, "We will also have you sign the Health Insurance Portability and Accountability Act, HIPAA, form that is a U.S. law designed to provide privacy standards to protect patient information. We need Ariella to sign an Assent Consent Form indicating that we have explained the diagnosis and treatment plan to her in age appropriate language."

After Susan translated, I explained that the chemotherapy drugs had all been tried and tested for over 30 years, were effective, and were proven to efficiently reduce immediate and long-term toxicities. Induction therapy lasts four and a half weeks, beginning with a three-day steroid prophase of intravenous methylprednisolone.

At this point in the conversation, I knew that Señora Colon must have been feeling overwhelmed, having received an enormous amount of emotionally draining information. If she was anything like others before her, I knew she would likely be unable to process additional information effectively, so I continued to write notes for her, and encouraged her to write down any questions.

The initial discussions with parents of new patients are unfathomably difficult—difficult for the doctor, difficult for the parents, and difficult for the patient. A fine line exists between too much and insufficient information. One must learn to read parents, determine their interest in comprehensive data, determine their level of understanding, and determine if they can process the information presented to them. Some families want to know everything, others not so much. Factor in the fact that the conversation doubles in length for non-English speaking families, and it is easy to appreciate a fatigue factor, not only for the parents, but for the physician and the interpreter as well. This isn't even including the massive volume of mandatory and exceedingly tedious paperwork that must be completed. Rules, regulations, HIPAA privacy, consents, assents, not to mention the complexity of the protocol, the chemotherapy, and information documents.

So, it was no surprise to us when Señora Colon started to fade. Her ability to listen and comprehend was understandably diminished, and she was left all alone to process, with her husband thousands of miles away. She had relatives in Washington Heights, an aunt and her family, but they were not available. Señora Colon began to well up. Danica moved close and offered her a tissue and water, gently holding her hand.

Señora Colon told us that she wanted to read the Spanish version of the documents and would sign the consents and forms, but for now she just wanted to return to her daughter's bedside. She was exhausted and she'd had enough.

Susan and Danica asked Señora Colon if she had any questions, but she did not. She sat quietly, with a glassy stare and facial expression of disbelief. One can only imagine what thoughts were swirling around in her mind. Would her daughter survive? Was it her fault that she'd become ill? How would she pay for the treatment? Would her son be all right or would he get leukemia as well? Where would she live? Where would her support come from? She was alone, and she needed her husband.

Danica and Susan promised Señora Colon that we would explain all of Ariella's results to her at each new phase of therapy. They promised that the entire team would do whatever possible for Ariella and the Colon family. "Our goal is to cure your daughter of this disease."

Lisa Jones handed the consents to Señora Colon and told her that we would leave them with her overnight and collect the signed forms in the morning. "Read them. If you have questions, write them down, and we will answer them all."

"*Gracias*," said Señora Colon. "I understand. *Gracias*."

Danica, Lisa, Señora Colon, and I then went into Ariella's hospital room. If the patient is over 8 years of age, we must obtain their assent prior to beginning therapy, explaining their diagnosis and treatment in an age-appropriate manner. I wanted Danica to speak directly to Ariella, explaining her diagnosis, treatment, and prognosis with kindness, competence, and compassion, demonstrating to Ariella and her family that they were in good hands. The first conversation is vital in establishing trust and rapport, and as Ariella's primary, it was crucial that Danica immediately prove herself to Ariella and Señora Colon.

Danica began in English, "Ariella, we want to tell you why you have not been feeling well, and why you are in the hospital. You have leukemia. It is a type of cancer that involves the bone marrow, or blood factory, and your bone marrow is not working normally; it is making abnormal cells that are called blasts."

Ariella, who was fully bilingual, responded in English, "Am I going to die? Do I have to stay in the hospital? I want to go home. I don't like it here. I'm afraid."

Danica instinctively moved close to Ariella's bedside, held her hand, and gently stroked her arm. "*Shhh*, don't be frightened. We're all here to help you and Mom."

Danica told Ariella that she would be fine; she needed treatment, but that we had excellent medicine called chemotherapy. She spoke about placing a PIC line for venous access and asked, "Can you swallow pills?"

"Yes, I think so."

"Good, that will make it easier for you. The chemotherapy is very effective. It will kill all of the leukemia blasts and allow your bone marrow blood factory to make good, normal, healthy cells. There are three kinds of blood cells made in the blood factory: red blood cells, platelets, and white blood cells. The red cells carry oxygen to our heart, brain, and other organs, the platelets prevent us from bleeding, and the white cells are the infection-fighting cells. If the red cell level is low, you will receive a red blood cell transfusion. If your platelet count is low, we can give you a transfusion of platelets. But, we cannot replace white blood cells, and if very low, you could develop fever and mouth sores and be susceptible to infection. You'll need antibiotics, and must stay in the hospital until your white blood cells recover to a safe level, usually about one to three weeks. I'm sorry."

"Am I going to lose my hair?" Ariella asked. "I had a friend in fourth grade who had leukemia, and he never came back to school. I think he was treated here, and he died. Am I going to die?"

"Ariella, there are many different types of leukemia, and each and every case is different, because no two patients are the same. From what we can tell about the type of leukemia that you have, we expect you to do well. We have excellent therapy, and we believe that you will do well and hopefully be cured."

"What about my hair?"

Ariella had thick, rich brown hair that flowed to the middle of her back. She loved her hair; it was a big part of her personality and even her identity—losing it would be traumatic.

"Yes, you will lose your hair, but it will grow back. If you want to wear a wig, you can get one that matches your own hair and the social workers can help you and your mom make arrangements."

Ariella rolled over in her hospital bed and covered her eyes, pulling the blanket over her head. She was finished listening to us.

Danica looked at me and raised her eyebrows as if to say, *What should we do now?*

It wasn't difficult to know that the conversation was over. Either Ariella was tired, frightened, or had heard enough about her future. The loss of her hair was the proverbial straw that broke the camel's back. Many young girls find this to be extremely difficult to navigate. It is less of an issue with boys, because a shaved head or a baseball cap is less conspicuous, but for the girls, it is a whole different matter. Señora Colon moved to the bed to try to comfort Ariella, but she would not be consoled. She wanted to be alone with her thoughts, grief, disbelief, and tears.

I told Mrs. Colon, "We need Ariella to sign the assent form indicating that we spoke to her about the leukemia, its treatment, and side effects." I told her that we would leave the paperwork and that Lisa Jones would be back in the morning to retrieve it. Mrs. Colon agreed, and we left the room.

We retreated to the team room on the fifth floor, a windowless space with a table in the center and blackboards affixed to the walls with five community computers. It was the room where rounds began and ended, and consults and patient decisions occurred. The team room also served as the working breakfast, lunch, and dinner room and the staff special occasion room. There was always food on the table—day old pizza, tasteless kosher cookies, or the ubiquitous bagel and cream cheese. Danica was despondent, believing she hadn't been able to reach Ariella.

I assured her she did a masterful job. "You spoke calmly, and delivered a simple, understandable message. Let's be certain we have remembered everything we need to get started with Ariella's treatment tomorrow morning. Did we schedule ENDO for the LP and PIC placement for tomorrow morning? Lisa and Danica, please write the chemo orders. Let's get the standard blood cultures, viral titers for herpes, CMV, varicella, and start Zosyn today."

"You know guys, I have a bad feeling about Ariella. I have never seen a patient with that degree of bone marrow necrosis at diagnosis. Not sure what it means; it makes me nervous. I hope I am wrong, let's get started and keep our fingers crossed. Are we all set to begin?"

"Yes," Danica replied. "I think we covered everything."

The next morning our team had to be divided to attend to a new patient who had been admitted during the night and mandated our immediate attention. Susan and I went to meet the Lefkowitz family while Danica and Lisa Jones went to Room 502 to complete Ariella Colon's enrollment into the study, answer questions, and collect the necessary documents we had left with Señora Colon the day before.

Danica and Lisa explained to Ariella and her mother the need to perform a diagnostic lumbar puncture while simultaneously administering cytarabine directly into the spinal fluid as prophylaxis to prevent the leukemia blast cells from invading the central nervous system. They mentioned that induction therapy begins with a three-day steroid prophase followed by a standard five-drug regimen including weekly IV vincristine, daily oral Decadron and intravenous doxorubicin, methotrexate, and PEG asparaginase. They told Ariella that we expected her to tolerate the therapy easily, we'd started Zosyn, an antibiotic to protect her from infections, and she would receive transfusions of blood and platelets.

In Spanish, Danica explained that the cytogenetics and molecular profiling from the bone marrow had not yet resulted. The duration of treatment lasts 25 to 26 months, is 90 percent effective with the vast majority of patients cured and returning to normal lives. She told Ariella and her mother that a bone marrow aspirate is performed after the four-week induction phase to determine initial response and remission status defined as less than 5 percent lymphoblasts, and MRD, less than 0.01 percent.

When Susan and I entered the room, the mood was somber.

Ariella and her mother were distraught, in disbelief, choking back tears, unable to speak. Their eyes told the story, there was nothing else to be said.

No Dogs Allowed

A riella's four-week induction phase went as was to be expected without untoward side effects. Ariella and her mother, on the other hand, remained in a continuous state of denial throughout, distant, non-communicative, and alone. I found it incredibly difficult to hold a meaningful conversation with Mrs. Colon. Meanwhile, Susan Garfield rotated off the oncology service and Danica Boyko joined the stem cell transplant group. My only remaining option was to use the hospital-provided Pacific interpreter service, which left my words lost in translation and my empathy unconveyed.

Señora Colon rarely left her daughter's room, ate barely a morsel, and slept in bed with Ariella rather than using the large, comfortable daybed available in her daughter's room. It was easy to see that she was exhausted. As Ariella made medical progress daily, her fever dissipating and blood counts recovering, so too did her psycho-emotional well-being improve. She began to smile and laugh, revealing an adorable personality beneath her grief and fear. Señora Colon, despite our inability to effectively converse, proved to be delightful, her disposition improving with her daughter's. We began communicating with hand signals and "*sí*" or "*no*." She was still afraid but was deeply grateful for the care her daughter was receiving.

As Ariella's uptick continued, we began to discuss discharge. It would not be simple or straightforward, however. Ariella had become ill in the Dominican Republic. When she had gone to the pediatrician there, he had ordered a blood test, which came back abnormal. By that evening, Señora

Colon and Ariella were already on a flight to JFK. Upon arrival, they hailed a cab to the pediatric emergency room at the Morgan Stanley Children's Hospital, and within 24 hours, they were under our care. The mother and daughter had only the clothes they were wearing, a change of underwear in a backpack, and a few dollars in their pocket. They had no insurance and no place to live except with an aunt in Washington Heights. In the ED, they were treated with respect. Ariella's blood count suggested probable leukemia, so she had been admitted to a private room. She was in not only the best children's hospital in New York, but one of the best in the country. They may have arrived without a plan to pay for Ariella's treatment, but there was no doubt that she would receive exceptional care.

Mrs. Colon informed Carol Vasquez, her social worker, that she had no place to go when Ariella was discharged; her Washington Heights relatives had indicated that there was no room at the inn. Carol suggested the Ronald McDonald House as a potential option, reminding us that Ariella had to remain hospitalized for a full 30 days in order to receive emergency Medicaid through the New York State Child Health Plus program.

The Ronald McDonald Houses are a global consortium of charitable homes that provide lodging for parents to stay close to their children who are sick and receiving medical treatment. The first house was opened in Philadelphia in 1974; today there are 368 houses across 64 countries. Although each operates independently, they share a common mission: to help families stay together through sickness, as they would in health.

The original New York Ronald McDonald House was incorporated in 1979, located on East 86th Street but was relocated to East 73rd and York in 1989. The new House is an 11-story facility with 95 private family suites. There are communal kitchens, dining facilities, activity rooms, media rooms, and meeting rooms, along with an extensive lineup of activities, events, tutoring, and wellness and support programs for guests. It is also the only House in the country to limit its occupancy to only the families of patients with cancer.

Charles Fowler the former Chief of Pediatric Surgery at Columbia and a close friend, asked me to join the board of the New York House, and I accepted. The experience was eye-opening. At my first meeting, held in a Midtown conference room of KPMG high above Sixth Avenue, I quickly recognized the seat of power and decision-making held by Rick O'Halloran, MD, Chief of the Pediatric Service at Memorial Sloan Kettering. As part of the board's executive committee, O'Halloran was involved in crucial decision-making, including the House's proximity to Memorial Sloan Kettering and its restriction to only serving the families of cancer patients. I learned that the operating budget, including mortgage and debt to run the House and support its programs, was between $8 and $10 million per year. The New York-based charity raised $15 million per year. I asked Barrett Stone, the local Board Chairman how the charity accounted for the $5–7 million not needed for operations.

"We invest the money in future needs, expansion, and special requests. Jack, why don't you give your investment report."

Jack, an investment banker and head of the charity's investment portfolio, proudly declared, "As of last week, we have $79 million in our accounts."

I was flabbergasted. $79 million. *Might there be an opportunity to expand and build a second New York City house in close proximity to Columbia?*, I wondered. I decided the prudent course of action would be to work back channels rather than go to the seat of power and let them know that I was questioning the status quo. I gathered data from the hospital administration to estimate potential usage and calculate the number of suites needed if we included non-cancer patients, which were accepted by every other RMH in the country, except the one in New York. I informed James Bergen and Ellen Stein, Chair of Pediatrics and the VP and Chief Operating Officer of the children's hospital, respectively, of my intentions and both supported my efforts. I prepared a presentation, made an appointment with Barrett Stone and Stan Schuster, Executive Director of the House, feeling optimistic. With a small fortune in the coffers, why shouldn't the board consider renovating a building in Washington Heights to serve as a satellite house?

The meeting did not go well.

Barrett told me that the board's policy was that any construction of a satellite house must be done in concert and partnership with the hospital. The hospital provides space or a building and renovates at their expense in accordance with RMH specifications. The House is then operated entirely by RMH staff.

"When the present house opened in 1989 on 73rd Street, two blocks from Memorial Sloan Kettering, did they buy the property and renovate at their expense?" I wondered.

"No, but things are different now."

"How so? What's different?"

"Well, then we didn't have this policy. Now we've decided to implement a new policy. So, you can see, there's really nothing we can do." Meeting adjourned.

I debriefed Bergen and Ellen, and neither was surprised. The hospital did not have available beds to offer and the cost of purchasing a suitable four- or five-story apartment building was prohibitive, thus there'd be nothing to renovate. Nothing more to discuss.

I soon resigned from the board, remaining on the mailing list where I was constantly solicited for money.

Several years later, I learned that the Ronald McDonald House of New York was planning a major renovation to the community space and adding six negative-pressure isolation rooms for severely compromised and stem cell transplant recipients. The cost? $15 million. Undoubtedly Rick O'Halloran at work. The audacity.

I called Barrett Stone and asked, "Tell me, Barrett, how does the decision to renovate the present house serve the interests of our children with cancer and their families?"

He had no answer other than to say the House needed an upgrade.

Despite my disdain, the RMH did serve a purpose, and at any given time, two or three Columbia patients were House residents. Its location was terribly inconvenient and required our families to commute crosstown via van between the hospital and East 73rd street. This was not optimal, especially for cancer patients, as the trip could take an hour each way in traffic. Meanwhile, Sloan Kettering patients walked across the street.

When Carol and Señora Colon visited the House, they were greeted warmly. They completed the application for admission, and Ariella was accepted as a resident upon discharge from the hospital. Prior to her release from Tower 5, Danica and I performed the day-32 bone marrow. There was no evidence of leukemia and the MRD was negative, a complete remission with final low-risk characteristics—great news.

The next phases of therapy went swimmingly. Ariella suffered a minor allergic reaction to asparaginase, which we were able to circumvent with premedication, but nothing serious. Danica followed Ariella as a primary patient, and her Spanish allowed for easy communication. Life at the RMH was going well; travel was not so onerous. Ariella participated in activities, gravitating to artwork and creating beautiful, mature watercolor paintings of her house in the Dominican Republic and the Caribbean Sea. Señora Colon was a delightful woman. In a hybrid mix of broken English and Spanish, she told us stories of her family and how beautiful and peaceful life had been at her home in the suburbs of Santo Domingo.

Danica and I were pleased with Ariella's progress, but one thing perplexed us—she never lost her hair. That was quite unusual. We questioned whether, despite being in remission with a negative MRD, the chemotherapy was truly effective and how deep the remission was. Shortly thereafter, about a year from diagnosis, we had our answer.

The treatment had betrayed Ariella. She developed fever, abdominal pain, and peripheral blasts, certain signs of relapse confirmed by a bone marrow aspirate. Señora Colon had told us that she sensed something awful was about to happen. She was right.

"Relapse" and "recurrence" are terrifying words—words that thrust cancer patients and their parents into a world of chaos, where the odds of cure dramatically decline and death is increasingly likely. The conversation with Mrs. Colon was difficult—virtually impossible, really. She expected the news, but that was of little help. Before she even entered the room on Irving-7, Señora Colon was fragile and crying. Thankfully, Danica was available, as was Daniella Cortez, a social worker, both of whom could speak to Señora Colon in her native language with kindness and compassion.

Danica told Mrs. Colon that Ariella's bone marrow was positive. "She's relapsed."

Screaming as she slid from her chair onto the floor, Señora Colon cried, "*¡No, no, no! ¡Dios mio! ¡Dios mio!*"

The conversation was soon over. We tried to be calm, to present a plan of hope, confidence, options, and potential new therapies, but Señora Colon heard nothing; her emotions and psyche were as broken as a vase, its pieces shattered everywhere. Ariella was admitted to the hospital where intensive therapy began anew.

The results of the recent relapsed marrow were perplexing. Whereas the original diagnostic marrow was acellular with normal cytogenetics, the current relapsed marrow had 60 percent blasts and the cytogenetics revealed a hypodiploid, karyotype-36 chromosomes.

Human genetic information is found in the 23 pairs of chromosomes, but the 23rd pair is special—the sex chromosomes, X and Y. Females have a pair of X chromosomes (46, XX), whereas males have one X and one Y chromosomes (46, XY). Leukemia blasts, like every other cell in every organ, bone, and blood cell have 46 chromosomes, a diploid modal number.

Ariella's leukemic blasts had 36 chromosomes, hypodiploid, or less than 46, an indication of aberrant genetic material and an ominous prognostic finding. A TP53 gene mutation was detected as well. The TP53 gene provides instructions for making a protein called tumor protein p53, which is a tumor suppressor that regulates cell division by preventing cells from proliferating in an uncontrolled way. It also regulates DNA repair. By stopping cells with mutated or damaged DNA from dividing, p53 helps prevent the development of tumors. Because p53 is essential for regulating DNA repair and cell division, it is essential to guard the genome. Because the leukemic blasts found in Ariella's bone marrow had a mutant, aberrant TP53, her leukemia was free to expand unchecked, without suppression.

Our leukemia doctors were puzzled. We questioned whether the new leukemia characteristics were de novo changes secondary to the chemotherapy, an unusual though well-known phenomenon, or whether Ariella's leukemia cells were evolving and self-selecting a resistant clonal change. The answer was speculative—hypothetical—it would never be answered. Regardless, it was a bad sign.

I walked into Ariella's room on Tower 5 to discuss options for new therapy. Danica was not able to join Lisa Jones and me for the discussion. We accessed the video interpreter, sub-optimal, but we needed a new set of consents and assents signed for the new protocol: Children's Oncology Group (COG) number AALL1331. The interpreter introduced himself as Pedro Alonzo. "*Buenos dias.*"

Señora Colon, in bed next to her daughter, was not interested in any discussion. She was withdrawn, teary, fearful, and non-communicative. It was déjà vu. In Spanish, she told Mr. Alonzo to tell the doctors that she just wanted to sign the documents.

"*¿Que otra opacion tengo?*" *What choice do I have?*

A profound observation, if not unique. How many times had I heard this same reluctant resignation from the parents of sick children as they attempted to come to terms with whatever unimaginable new reality lay before them? It is heartbreaking for a parent to realize that they are powerless in the face of disease, that they cannot protect their child. The happiness of any parent is tied inextricably to their child's well-being. A cancer diagnosis, and especially a cancer resurgence, can be as brutally painful for a parent as it is for a child.

Ariella received an intensive five-drug re-induction therapy with the addition of a new targeted immunotherapeutic agent, BLINCYTO, which had been proven to improve survival rates significantly in patients similar to Ariella. The downside was that, as with many oncological advances, weighty toxicity exists, most notably cytokine release syndrome, and neurological complications. To mitigate some of these adverse side effects—which include fever, headache, nausea, asthenia or more serious effects like hypotension, liver damage, disseminated intravascular coagulation, and excessive internal bleeding—Ariella received premedication with dexamethasone, Benadryl, and Tylenol.

Ariella did well. She suffered no untoward side effects, with one exception—she finally lost her hair. Danica and I were optimistic; we reasoned that the depth of chemotherapy now was deep and effective. Ariella, on the other hand, was crushed. Her beautiful, thick, flowing dark hair was her identity and now it was gone, probably forever. She was inconsolable. The social workers arranged for her to have a custom-made wig crafted by an expensive hair boutique; Hope & Heroes paid the cost, no questions asked. Katherine from the Andrew de Silva Salon came to the children's hospital for a fitting, and by the time they'd found just the right fit, Ariella looked exquisite. Her smile reached from ear to ear; it was a joyful day.

The day of Ariella's bone marrow exam, the air was thick and anxiety was high. The results of this exam would determine Ariella's uncertain future. The results were devastating: 60 percent blasts—no response whatsoever. There was no need for MRD testing; the results were obvious.

I dreaded having to relay the bad news to Señora Colon as she was already so fragile. She was waiting nervously when we entered Ariella's room and immediately read the disappointment written on our faces; our eyes foretold the bad news. We escorted Señora Colon to the meditation room, but before we even sat down, she was sobbing uncontrollably. I felt fortunate that Danica was available. It was imperative that Señora Colon be able to not only hear the news in her native tongue but from a sensitive source— someone with whom she had an established connection. Danica explained that leukemia blasts represented the majority of the marrow cells and that the recently completed treatment did not accomplish what we had hoped. We believed that Señora Colon heard and understood that much of the conversation but probably not much more.

She repeated over and over, "Please help my daughter! Don't let her die! Help her! Help her!"

Though the present outlook was grim and the odds were mounting, we still had tools in our toolbox. Danica mentioned that there was an exciting new treatment available for patients with refractory ALL, CAR-T cell therapy followed by an allogeneic stem cell transplant. She informed Señora Colon that we had already spoken to Dr. Krishana who runs the CAR-T program and he had indicated that Ariella would be an excellent candidate, though he suggested additional chemotherapy as a bridge. We decided to employ Inotuzumab ozogamicin, BESPONSA, an antibody drug-conjugate that consists of a humanized monoclonal antibody against CD22 on the surface of the blast cells, linked to a cytotoxic agent, ozogamicin, an anti-tumor antibiotic. It is amenable to outpatient administration, given as a single agent once a week for three weeks and may be repeated if efficacy is demonstrated.

We discharged Ariella, who returned to a homecoming celebration at the Ronald McDonald House. The other families embraced Ariella and Mrs. Colon; they were a fraternity, a family bonded by experience, although one that none of them would have willingly joined. Like it or not, they were in this together, sharing the triumphs and the tragedies, sharing hope, despair, joy, grief, and suffering. That night in the RMH community room, the residents had a welcome home party for Ariella, who looked beautiful in her new wig. The kitchen staff prepared her favorite dish, rice and beans with chicken fajitas. As the kids played board games and sang songs, Mrs.

Colon told several of the other parents the disquieting news that Ariella's latest bone marrow results were not good, she continued to have active leukemia. One of the Sloan Kettering mothers, whose four-year-old son had neuroblastoma, said, "We will pray for you."

"*Gracias.*"

Ariella received an outpatient course of BESPONSA, but the repeat bone marrow revealed that 70 percent of the blasts were resistant—disappointing but not the end of the world. We had more modalities such as CAR-T cell therapy, a type of ingenious treatment developed in 1989 by Drs. Yoshikazu Kuwana of Japan and Zelig Eshhar of Israel, which was first used in the United States by Carl June and his colleagues at the University of Pennsylvania. In principle, a patient's immune T-cells are engineered in the laboratory by inserting a special receptor gene, a chimeric antigen receptor (CAR), which binds to a certain protein on the patient's cancer cells. Millions of patient-specific CAR-T cells are grown and then reinfused intravenously. The CAR-T cells are able to bind to the CD19 antigen on the leukemia cells, become activated, proliferate, become cytotoxic, and kill them. It's like a living drug against cancer cells. For safety, CAR-T cells are derived to be specific to a tumor antigen that is not expressed on healthy cells. Several commercial laboratories have FDA approval to manufacture CAR-T cells; at Columbia, Dr. Krishana and his team use a Novartis product, Tisagenlecleucel, KYMRIAH. We would try this next.

The KYMRIAH infusion was uneventful. Ariella tolerated it well, with only minor symptoms of fever and chills, relieved by an anti-inflammatory agent. Clinically, Ariella improved. Her bone pain decreased, and she experienced less fatigue and improved energy. Although her peripheral counts stabilized, the bone marrow test again showed blasts—95 percent. Our options were diminishing. To date, she had received standard acute lymphoblastic leukemia induction, second- and third-attempt re-induction with BLINCYTO and BESPONSA, respectively, followed by CAR-T cell therapy, all of which had failed. The possibility of meaningful survival with any positive quality of life was virtually nil. The cost of Ariella's fully loaded treatment was astronomical, between hospitalization, medication, professional fees, etc., it approximated $1 million. The expense of the KY-MRIAH alone was $400,000.

The mood at the RMH was somber. Far too often, the patient and family community on East 73rd Street had to somehow come to terms with the impending loss of one of their own. For all of us, that loss is personal; it indicates a failure, even knowing that we had done absolutely everything that we could. The overarching sentiment shared by all was that fear today was a more powerful emotion than tomorrow's grief. Such is the scourge of childhood cancer.

We asked Señora Colon if it were possible for her husband to be with her and Ariella. She informed us that she had already asked him to come to New York and that he would arrive in a few days.

Ariella and her parents took the RMH shuttle from the tony Upper East Side to the working-class neighborhood of Washington Heights. The luxury high-rise apartments and expensive restaurants and shops on Third Avenue were replaced by bodegas, housing projects, and discount liquor stores—life's inequities made almost comically obvious.

When they arrived back at the Irving Pavilion, Ariella said hello to the security guard in the lobby, who greeted the Colon family with a smile, handed them hospital passes, and waved them through. They took the elevator to 7. Ariella was joyful and anxious to introduce her father, who was embarrassed by all the fuss, to Michah and Carla at the front desk; to Yasmin, the phlebotomist; to her favorite nurses, Cathy and May; to Carol Vasquez, her social worker; to Misty Carlson, the acupuncturist; and to Rosalia, one of the child-life specialists.

"Everyone, this is my dad!" Ariella proudly proclaimed.

After the introductions, she had her PORT accessed and blood drawn. Her blood count was terrible—50 percent blasts, platelets at 22,000, and hemoglobin at 6.8 g/dl. She needed transfusions of packed red blood cells and platelets. It would be a long day in clinic.

Señor and Señora Colon and I retreated to one of the consultation rooms, where we were joined by Jane Stark, a leukemia team nurse practitioner. Ariella slept in one of the large blue lounge chairs, drowsy from the Benadryl premedication for her blood and platelet transfusions. Mr. Colon was a large man, probably close to 250 pounds, with thinning black-gray hair, and an affable smile. Although obviously exhausted from travel, it was equally clear that he was glad to be with his wife and daughter in New York. Danica was unavailable, so we scheduled an in-person Spanish translator, Rodrigo Perez. The Colons sat next to each other on the bench seat, holding hands, while Mary, Rodrigo, and I sat in chairs facing them. Together, we had difficult decisions to make.

"Mr. and Mrs. Colon, unfortunately and surprisingly the CAR-T cell therapy was not effective. Ariella's marrow remains totally replaced by leukemia blasts."

I waited for Rodrigo to translate, but before he finished Señora Colon began to cry, "No, no! How could this be? We have done everything—nothing works. Please don't let our daughter die."

As Señora Colon wept, Señor Colon was speechless, frozen as a deer in headlights. He was silent as he held his wife tenderly, tight to his body.

I told the Colons that there were two paths forward. The first, continued ultra-aggressive therapy, that frankly had little chance of being effective; or a palliative approach, predicated on supportive care measures, pain management, perhaps a return to the Dominican Republic, time with family and friends, and as much time as possible out of the hospital. Continued treatment would require long hospitalizations, transfusions, risk of infections, and other complications; I reiterated further chemotherapy had little chance of meaningful success.

The Colons faced Sophie's Choice. The decision was impossible to make, and I wondered what I would have done. It is a question that is unanswerable, a decision that can only be made in the moment, a decision for which one can never prepare. Certainly, I was not prepared to make such a decision, not now or any time soon. Thus, when Señor Colon asked me what I would do, I answered, "Please forgive me. I'm sorry, but I do not have the solution."

I told them through the interpreter that there was no correct answer. It is personal and based on family beliefs, culture, faith, and importantly, their tolerance and the tolerance of their child to be able to endure long hospital stays, pain, and suffering.

I suggested that they take some time to decide. They should go back to the RMH and discuss things with Ariella. They agreed that Ariella should be included in the decision, however painful.

It was clear that Ariella's death was imminent, measured in months. If the Colons wanted treatment, she would spend the majority of her remaining days in the hospital. If the Colons selected palliative, supportive care, her life would be shorter, but the quality of her days would be significantly improved, perhaps including a return to the Dominican Republic.

Ariella and her parents returned the next day. Danica was available to participate in the conversation. She adroitly asked Ariella, "Did you discuss with your parents what you want to do next?"

Ariella answered in English, "Yes. I really want to go home to see my family and friends in the Dominican Republic, but my parents want me to get treatment. We compromised; I'll take more chemo, but when it is over, they said we can go to the DR to visit."

"That seems fair—a good plan."

"I have a question. I would really like a dog. Can I get a puppy? Please!"

"We'll look into the puppy. We need to speak to the people at RMH to see if they have a policy."

Ariella seemed happy, momentarily pacified—a child unable to internalize the scope of her illness.

"Are you ready to be admitted today?"

The Colons, despite their limited English, understood the entire conversation and agreed that Ariella should be admitted that day. They supported the idea of the puppy if the House agreed, and, like most parents, would have done anything to see their daughter happy. We administered Clofarabine, Cytoxan, and Etoposide and hoped for bone marrow aplasia. If attained, the stem cell transplant team indicated they would do a transplant. Ariella had a perfectly matched, unrelated donor who already consented, and was available to donate stem cells when called. She tolerated the regimen without significant side effects. On the positive side, her bone pain improved and her peripheral blood counts were extremely low. We were guardedly optimistic.

The morning of the next bone marrow exam, Ali Mahesh, Chief of Hematopathology, expedited his interpretation: aplastic, no normal hematopoiesis, necrotic, however, the only cells observed are clusters of leukemia blasts. "This kid cannot catch a break."

Danica and I entered Ariella's room, which was spotlessly clean—bed made, towels folded, books, games, and toys all neatly in place, floor and bathroom sparkling. Mrs. Colon, as always, was in bed with her daughter, stroking her back and arms; Señor Colon stood and greeted us.

Ariella insisted on participating in discussions. She was clearly involved in decision-making; it was her life after all. Danica spoke directly to Ariella and told her that her marrow was empty—a good sign. She did not mention the blast-cell clusters but told her that we wanted to repeat the marrow in two weeks. The follow-up marrow was no better in terms of necrosis and blasts. Extensive discussions ensued in an attempt to establish goals of care. Señora Colon, unable to confront reality, was exhausted and emotionally spent in a trance-like inertia, barely able to communicate her thoughts. Her exhaustion was no match for fear: fear of losing her daughter, fear of the unknown, fear of death. Mr. Colon remained distant, listening without asking questions, unable to provide any visible support to either his wife or daughter.

Despite her young age, Ariella was her family's source of strength. She understood the dire circumstances, understood that the chemo was ineffective, and she was tired and frustrated. She wanted a puppy, and she wanted to return to her beautiful home in the Dominican Republic. She informed her parents in no uncertain terms, "I'm done, no more."

The family needed time—time to talk, time to think, time to plan, time to be together; they sheltered in their room at the RMH—no puppies allowed, house rules. Señora Colon contacted Carol Vasquez. "We would like to go home; can you help us make arrangements?"

Carol, working with Dan Todd, Executive Director of Hope & Heroes, went into overdrive to make travel arrangements, airline tickets, ground transportation, everything. Danica spoke to a physician at the children's hospital in Santo Domingo about Ariella and arranged for her to receive blood transfusions, antibiotics, and pain medication, if needed. The evening before departure, with luggage packed and placed at the door of their suite at the RMH, Ariella developed a fever of 103 degrees. She arrived at the emergency department with her white blood cell counts virtually non-existent, at great risk for an overwhelming infection. She was admitted to Tower 5. Their plans dashed, Ariella and her parents were devastated, realizing that their daughter's dream of going home was over.

Ariella was sick—her blood cultures positive for Klebsiella. Antibiotics were altered to treat this unwanted bacterial invader, not easy in the absence of infection fighting white blood cells. When Ariella's count did rise, it did so with a vengeance—leukemia blasts, expanding the bone marrow cavity and causing severe back and extremity pain. She then developed abdominal pain, cramps, and diarrhea; Clostridium dificil, an opportunistic organism that attacks the gut, was the culprit.

Ariella was miserable, in pain, suffering. Mr. and Mrs. Colon were in shock. Visits to the room became increasingly uncomfortable as we had nothing positive to say and the family was exhausted from hearing more bad news. Always polite, the Colons simply had nothing to say, no questions to ask. They acknowledged our presence and remained unquestionably grateful for our efforts, but there were no words. Terminal leukemia in its final stages is relentless, akin to a slow march toward a certain outcome: death.

Unfortunately, Ariella's problems persisted. She developed severe headaches and ptosis of her right eye. The differential diagnoses, central nervous system leukemia versus an intracranial hemorrhage, were both terrible. An emergency MRI of her brain revealed the former. When we explained the results to Ariella and her parents, she screamed, "No more spinal taps! Please, please, I beg you! No more!"

Mrs. Colon, her voice barely audible, asked, "Is there an alternative to the lumbar punctures?"

"Yes. We should be able to arrange for palliative radiation treatments to her head, and we can add Decadron to reduce brain swelling. I'll call Dr. Dr. Kennedy to set it up."

"*Gracias, gracias*—thank you, thank you."

Danica Boyko, not one to leave a stone unturned, suggested Venetoclax, an oral agent, as a rational drug for Ariella. It would be used in combination with Azacytidine, Venetoclax targets the anti-apoptotic protein, Bcl-2, linked to chemotherapy resistance in patients with hypodiploid mutated TP53—experimental for sure, but worth a try. In addition, the possibility existed that new drugs might—just might—lessen her unimaginable pain temporarily.

Danica and I entered the room wearing gowns, masks, and gloves to prevent the spread of the C. dificil. Ariella was asleep, sedated from the pain medication, with a continuous infusion of Ketamine and PCA, patient-controlled analgesia, with Dilaudid intravenously, a temporary relief for her pain. Mrs. Colon, as always, was in bed with her daughter, stroking her legs and back, and caressing her bald, beautiful head. The pain she experienced had many tentacles, anger at the injustice of losing her daughter, helplessness at being unable to reverse the inevitable, concern about how she and her husband could continue living without Ariella, and deep, unimaginable sadness, like nothing experienced before. Mr. Colon, on the other hand, seemed numb, standing in the corner and smiling from the corner of his mouth to acknowledge our presence.

Danica, in Spanish, explained the possibility of administering a new drug combination: Azacytidine IV and Venetoclax orally. She told the Colons that it was safe for us to begin today, and that it had the potential for mitigating Ariella's pain. Our hope was to buy time and extend life, if possible—nothing more. They understood, agreed with the plan, and thanked us for trying.

The chemotherapy had the desired effect—less pain, control of the bacterial sepsis, resolution of gastrointestinal symptoms, and the successful management of the central nervous system disease.

The pain and palliative care team changed her analgesia to an oral Oxycodone plus Fentanyl patches. Ariella was discharged to the RMH, with scheduled daily visits to Irving-7 for counts, hydration, transfusions, and whatever else she needed.

The ambulatory sojourn was short-lived, lasting only two days. Ariella's fever, severe pain, and hypotension returned, even more debilitating than before. A CT scan of Ariella's entire body revealed the cruelty of terminal leukemia, extensive bone destruction in her spine, extremities, pelvis, and skull—the etiology of her unrelenting pain. She also had hypodense lesions in her liver compatible with a disseminated fungal infection, so we began Ambisome, an antifungal drug. Pain meds were reintroduced. Ariella, thankfully heavily sedated, rested peacefully. When she stirred, she seemed agitated and uncomfortable, so the dosages were increased to alleviate her symptoms, anxiety, and pain.

Discussions with the family were brief, as the Colons recognized their daughter's plight. Danica and I asked them to join us in the meditation room to review Ariella's condition, answer questions, and obtain the obligatory DNI/DNR (do not intubate/do not resuscitate) orders and consents. Speaking slowly, calmly, and compassionately in Spanish, Danica detailed Ariella's status and how we would address each issue on the problem list; fulminant leukemia, bacterial and fungal sepsis, and unremitting pain were the issues of significance. She explained our focus was pain management and comfort.

I informed the Colons that we would discontinue the Venetoclax and Azacytidine and instead begin Nivolumab, a type of cancer immunotherapy that targets immune checkpoints to stimulate an immune response against the leukemia or cancer cells. I explained that the drug was given orally, and we anticipated no adverse effects or downside. I told them that despite the introduction of Nivolumab, our anticipation of Ariella's death had not changed. They agreed.

Danica continued in Spanish, translating my comments and began to describe the need for DNI/DNR. Señora Colon, weeping continuously and quietly, did not speak and seemed incapable of sharing thoughts or asking questions. Mr. Colon held her tightly and tenderly, offering tissues as he began to cry as well.

In Spanish, Mr. Colon said, "We understand. We agree, of course. We pray for peace; we don't want Ariella to suffer or be in pain."

The room was quiet with everyone deep in personal reflection. There was nothing else to say except, "We are so sorry."

"*Gracias.* Thank you, doctor."

The days prior to her death, Ariella deteriorated neurologically, experiencing increased somnolence and respiratory distress. The Ketamine and Dilaudid were increased. She passed away peacefully with her mother in her bed, stroking her back, caressing her head, and kissing her tenderly.

Mrs. Colon, in that moment, lost part of her being, her essence, her reason for living; if conceivable, she would have permanently affixed their bodies together, never leaving Ariella's side. There was no bottom to her despair. I had no doubt that, if she could have sacrificed her own life for Ariella's, she would have.

Mrs. Colon refused to allow the five Tower nurses to clean and prepare Ariella for the morgue. She was hysterical. Mr. Colon attempted to console his wife, but it was not possible. She was incapable of saying goodbye. The nurses and staff respected her space, and no one entered the room. After what seemed like an eternity, Mr. and Mrs. Colon exited the hospital room, their personal effects packed, said brief goodbyes, and abruptly left.

Ariella was then prepared for her final trip to the Dominican Republic.

MARK ALAN NIEMAN

Natural Killer Cells

My iPhone vibrated in my pocket. "Yes, what's up?"

"We have a new consult—a two-year-old female with an abnormal count. The peripheral flow is pending; it should be resulted within the hour. Are you available to meet with me, review the chart, and meet the patient and family?"

"Of course," I said. "I'm about done with clinic patients. I'll meet you in the Tower 5 team room in an hour."

Chaya Lefkowitz's case was fascinating, if infuriatingly opaque. Since infancy, she had been followed by Dr. Linda Gerald, the former chief of pediatric rheumatology and immunology, who remained unclear on a comprehensive prognosis. Dr. Gerald's research and evaluations into Chaya's condition had been exhaustive, and yet, Chaya's complicated medical history left more questions open than resolved. She suffered from episodes of recurrent high fever associated with severe pancytopenia and bona fide bacterial infections. Linda directed an extensive evaluation investigating all known existing conditions compatible with Chaya's symptoms; she consulted Wynne Kang from molecular genetics, recognizing that there are over 300 genetic defects that can cause immunodeficiency disorders; she consulted colleagues at Boston Children's Hospital, Children's Hospital of Philadelphia, as well as Texas and Cincinnati Children's Hospitals. Still, Chaya's underlying condition remained elusive.

Unable to identify a root cause, Linda empirically treated Chaya with glucocorticoids and monthly infusions of serum immunoglobulins and antibiotics. The regimen mitigated the recurring episodes, but it did not prevent symptom recurrence. The case was baffling, frustrating.

Linda Gerald had spent the entirety of her career at Columbia; she'd completed her residency at Columbia Presbyterian and never left. She trained in pediatric rheumatology with Neil Margolis, the first division chief and program director at the then–Babies Hospital, a founding member of the specialty sub-board for the American Board of Pediatrics, and the author of the magnum opus in pediatric rheumatology. I knew Neil and recall being a young attending physician at Babies in the late 1970s, asking him to do a consult on a patient.

Despite his idiosyncratic personality, Neil was a phenomenal doctor and an incredible mentor to Linda Gerald before his untimely and painful death from colon cancer. Linda succeeded Neil, and has proven herself to be a superb clinician, though an inadequate division director and leader. She was terrible at managing divisional finances and rarely complied with the requisite responsibilities imposed by the hospital and Columbia University Medical Center. Donald Colbert, Chair of Pediatrics, demoted and unsuccessfully attempted to fire her; however, her husband, Alan Jonathan, an MD, PhD, tenured professor, teacher, and scientist extraordinaire, threatened to leave Columbia if she were terminated. Dean Sterngold intervened, Jonathan prevailed, and Linda joined the division of rheumatology in the department of medicine and continues to see patients.

Having filled me in on this background, Charlie Bradley, seated at a computer checking results, said, "It's positive—the peripheral flow is positive."

Together, we reviewed Chaya's complicated history, multiple hospital admissions, page after page of outpatient visits, hundreds of laboratory results, consult reports from experts around the country all facilitated by the electronic medical record. Chaya's charts included a bone marrow aspirate and biopsy report from the Dana-Farber Cancer Center in Boston. It had been obtained three months earlier and was normal, negative, no evidence of leukemia. Confounding the clinical picture was the fact that Chaya had received high-dose steroids therapeutically for management of exacerbations and continued on low-dose prednisone prophylactically. Steroids, as a single agent, suppress leukemia cell proliferation and may temporarily induce a complete remission.

Charlie and I entered Room 516 and introduced ourselves to Mr. Lefkowitz. "I'm Dr. Weiner, and this is Dr. Bradley. Good to meet you."

"Dr. Weiner, I've been expecting you." He raised a finger to his lips indicating please be quiet. "Chaya is asleep, can we speak outside?"

We sat in the alcove across from Chaya's room. Mr. Lefkowitz was an Orthodox man, not Hasidic. He had prematurely gray hair, a short, groomed beard, wire-frame gold glasses, and a *yarmulke* atop his head. He wore the obligatory black pants, white shirt, and black shoes with the laces untied, but he seemed somehow more contemporary, perhaps because the family lived in Riverdale, an integrated, multicultural, multi-religious community, rather than in an enclave in Williamsburg or Borough Park in Brooklyn, or Monsey. It was immediately apparent that Mr. Lefkowitz was incredibly intelligent. He had taken the time to research every aspect of his daughter's medical history and condition and was almost encyclopedic in his knowledge of her case. His comprehension of NK cells and perforin function in health and disease was expansive. He was logical, thoughtful, and asked pointed questions, even if we were unable to provide readily apparent answers. He already knew the peripheral flow was consistent with leukemia, and he reminded us that Chaya had had a bone marrow test several months earlier and it had been normal. He informed us that she had not been on steroids at the time, indicating his understanding that prednisone is a drug used to treat leukemia.

I told him that we needed to repeat the bone marrow and do a diagnostic lumbar puncture with intrathecal cytarabine.

"I'll consent to the marrow and spinal tap, but no medicine. Chaya is not like other patients, she is unique unto herself," Mr. Lefkowitz said.

We agreed. "But let's get the marrow and LP behind us. We'll schedule it for tomorrow morning in the procedure room under anesthesia."

The following morning, both procedures went smoothly. I explained the results to Mr. Lefkowitz and told him the bone marrow flow cytometry and morphology confirmed acute lymphoblastic leukemia—straightforward, no ambiguity, no doubt. I explained that there were no adverse biomarkers, hyperdiploid, favorable cytogenetics, RUNX1 mutation positive as well—another good prognosis indicator; the cerebrospinal fluid was devoid of leukemia, no evidence of CNS involvement.

"Dr. Weiner, I have no doubt you're correct that Chaya has leukemia," said Mr. Lefkowitz. "I was aware that patients with NK cell mutations had an increased risk of leukemia, but before we begin treatment, I need your assistance. I want to contact the people in Boston and Cincinnati, have them review the bone marrow material, and offer an opinion."

I readily agreed.

"I'll get you the names and addresses. Can you send the bone marrow slides and reports to Boston Children's and Cincinnati Children's? Also, can you ask Dr. Greene if he would see Chaya and speak to us as well?"

"Dr. Greene is aware and will be by this afternoon. As soon as you have the addresses for us, we will Fed Ex overnight the slides and reports," I said. "We've also asked Linda Gerald to join us for a conversation. Does 3 this afternoon work? Is your wife available, would she like to join the conversation?"

Appointed in July 2018, Evan Greene is the new Chairman of Pediatrics at Columbia and Pediatrician in Chief at New York Presbyterian. He is an internationally renowned scientist, recently elected to the prestigious National Academy of Science, and has received numerous accolades for his discovery and innovation in his area of expertise, natural killer cells. The first time I met him, several months before his start date, was at a meeting with the three other vice chairs of the department: Joel Peters, Sydney

Gold, and Rob Porter. Evan introduced himself, but rather than detail his research and career, he told us that he was a New Yorker, raised in Great Neck, Long Island. He told us that his father, a dentist, had passed away suddenly, and that his mother was still alive and working as a high school guidance counselor. Evan had gone to Brown for undergrad and medical school, and had been on the swim team. He told us about his wife Katie, a nurse, whom he'd met at CHOP, and with whom he had three daughters. The conversation was relaxed and genuine; it was clear that Evan saw himself first and foremost as a family man, rather than someone defined by his professional accomplishments. I liked him immediately.

Returning to Room 516 for our 3 p.m. conversation, I found both Mr. and Mrs. Lefkowitz and one of Chaya's grandfathers by her bedside. "Dr. Greene messaged that he is on his way," I said. "Unfortunately, there are no conference or meeting rooms on the floor that will accommodate the group; Dr. Greene attracts a crowd."

I suggested we use the community area near the playroom. It had ample room and plenty of chairs. When we arrived, Linda and Evan were already there. Linda introduced Evan Greene, salutations were offered, and everyone made themselves comfortable. Evan and Linda had already spoken about Chaya, and he had reviewed her medical record and history—he was up to speed. Evan told Chaya's parents that he agreed with the diagnosis of natural killer cell deficiency and the management invoked by Dr. Gerald, and most importantly, he concurred with the diagnosis of acute lymphoblastic leukemia. He told Mr. and Mrs. Lefkowitz that he had taken the liberty of speaking with his colleagues in Boston and Cincinnati who had advised him to treat the leukemia.

Mr. Lefkowitz thanked Dr. Greene, resigned to the diagnosis of B-cell ALL, and consented to begin treatment. He signed the necessary consent forms and HIPAA documents; treatment would begin the next morning.

After Chaya's parents left, Evan began a diatribe about NK cells, their discovery, and their recognition as an integral component of the immune system, function, and disease states. No one knew more about natural killer cells than he. When Evan was on the faculty at CHOP in Philadelphia, he had a State of Pennsylvania vanity license plate: NK CELL. He mentioned to the assembled group of trainees and students that Mark Nieman, a patient whom I had cared for 30 years before, had an undiagnosed primary immunodeficiency disease, but, in retrospect, had a perforin deficiency and dysfunctional NK cells.

I recall Mark Nieman and his parents, Frank and Madeline—my goodness, what memories.

The Niemans epitomized young, hip, progressive New Yorkers. Recently married, they lived in a new luxury building on the Upper East Side of Manhattan, with views of the city skyline, the Empire State Building, and Rockefeller Center. Madeline was only 21 years old and newly graduated from New York University. She was radiant with long, flowing dirty blond hair, a perpetual smile, and sharp outfits. Frank, smitten with his new bride, was a handsome, dark-haired man. They were more than elated when Mark was born, a beautiful, healthy, robust baby boy. They were a handsome threesome, proud and bursting with joy. Frank and Madeline could not have been happier.

The Niemans spent Mark's first summer in Southampton, an escape from the stifling heat of the city. Their rental house—a quaint, two-story, weather-shingled gem with a white wrap-around front porch, manicured gardens, and a swing set in the backyard—was perfectly located within walking distance of the village. It was an idyllic summer set up for a young family of three. Their days were filled with stroller rides to the village and visits to the Town Beach to play in the sand, Mark sat happily in his navy blue Bugaboo, while Frank and Madeline window-shopped at Saks and the overpriced boutiques.

One balmy evening, as Madeline bathed Mark in the kitchen sink, a cool Atlantic Ocean breeze tempering the heat of day, she noticed that Mark felt feverish. When his temperature read 104 degrees, she called her pediatrician, Irwin Moskowitz. He instructed Frank and Madeline to give Mark ibuprofen, then immediately get in the car and go to the emergency room at Mt. Sinai Hospital. "I'll meet you there."

Dr. Moskowitz graduated first in his class at Physicians & Surgeons of Columbia University and trained as a general pediatrician and pediatric endocrinologist at Babies Hospital. During WWII, he'd volunteered for the army and served in North Africa. After completing his military service, he entered the private practice of pediatrics in Manhattan and became a major figure in the Department of Pediatrics of Mt. Sinai Hospital. He was considered by all who interacted with him—patients, families, and colleagues—to be the foremost pediatrician, not only on the staff of Mt. Sinai, but in all of New York City.

In the emergency room, Mark appeared very ill. He was jaundiced with a high fever, rapid heart rate, and an enlarged liver and spleen. Blood work revealed pancytopenia, elevated bilirubin, and elevated liver transaminases; an abdominal ultrasound demonstrated an enlarged liver and spleen. Moskowitz admitted Mark to a single room on Falk 3, the private pediatric floor. Unlike Babies Hospital at Columbia where all patients were aggregated by age rather than by their ability to pay, Mt. Sinai's pediatric inpatient units were segregated socioeconomically—insurance and private versus Medicaid and charity care.

Moskowitz suspected liver disease and blocked bile ducts, perhaps caused by a viral infection. He asked Michael Field, a distinguished senior clinician and liver expert, to consult and perform a liver biopsy, which resulted with nonspecific changes—the biliary system was normal.

Mark completed an empiric two-week course of antibiotics; his fever abated and blood counts recovered, and he was discharged with a presumptive diagnosis of viral-induced hepatitis. The Niemans, although perplexed as to the etiology of the illness, were nevertheless relieved and thrilled to be going home with their son. Life continued as before, and Frank resumed work as a diamond dealer, manufacturer of fine jewelry, and landlord on 47th Street between 5th and 6th Avenue—the jewelry district.

For a time, Mark was well . . . until he was not. At 18 months old, he became ill again with identical symptoms, identical spectrum of disease, and identical treatment. He was soon discharged, home and well.

For six months, life resumed as normal. Mark, now two years old, was an adorable toddler, full of joy and energy. He appeared perfectly healthy and normal until, seemingly out of nowhere, he became ill a third time. He had identical symptoms, identical spectrum of disease. Frank and Madeline questioned Moskowitz. "Irwin, something's wrong here. This is not normal—something's wrong."

Moskowitz, without ego when it came to the well-being of his patients, asked Frank Siegal, an allergist and immunologist, to see Mark. Although thorough, kind, and sympathetic, he was not able to provide appropriate guidance. The field of immunology was in a nascent phase with little concrete information, descriptive in nature with little in the way of therapeutics. Dr. Siegal was able to conclude, however, that dysfunction of the immune system was possible—probable even—but exactly what the defect might be was highly speculative.

The spectrum of Mark's illness changed and followed a reproducible pattern—a roller coaster of ups and downs. Three to four times each year, he was hospitalized with unrelenting fever and pneumonia. He was quite ill, requiring oxygen, and often spent days on end in intensive care. But he always miraculously improved. He was a unique patient on the pediatric service at Mt. Sinai. Others had asthma, diabetes, leukemia, sickle cell anemia, and hemophilia, others were admitted for elective surgery. No one had repeated infections secondary to an immune system problem— no one. Between infectious episodes, he seemed fine with no hint of illness. He enjoyed playdates, took swimming lessons, went to Bill-Dave day camp. Frank and Madeline adjusted to a perplexing routine, a quarterly visit to the Falk Pavilion. It was troubling, but they made their peace with it—after all, Mark always got better.

Madeline and Frank had a very difficult decision to make. They desperately wanted another child and had always envisioned a family of two, perhaps three, children; however, given Mark's health, they were worried. Would another child suffer the same illness as Mark? They had no idea whether his condition was genetic or hereditary and they worried about their ability to manage a new baby. They consulted several experts. Drs. Jerry Tannenbaum, Chair of Pediatrics, and Lee Smith, Director of Genetics at Mt. Sinai, both world class experts, told the Niemans that there was no evidence to indicate that Mark's condition was hereditary. They mapped an extensive family tree, yet nowhere could they find a family member with symptoms similar to Mark's. Tannenbaum believed his illness was random, but there was a caveat. He told them that, in truth, they just did not know for certain.

Pregnancy was joyful for Madeline. She felt well, glowing, healthy. Mark was also thrilled, ecstatic to have a younger brother or sister. Frank, in a word, was great—he was happy and his business was booming. Madeline delivered a beautiful, apparently healthy baby girl, whom they named Debbie. However, it was soon evident that something was not right. Debbie's eyes failed to track, she did not respond to noise, and she sucked weakly. Moskowitz advised, "Give it some time. See what develops. It is too early to draw conclusions."

Mark had another episode of fever and pneumonia, which required hospitalization, and Madeline stayed at his side for three weeks. Frank worked a few hours in the morning, then joined Madeline and Mark in the Falk Pavilion in the afternoon. At night, he was too tired to dote over Debbie, who was cared for by a nurse. As always, Mark recovered with antibiotics, oxygen, and rest—nothing unusual—but Debbie presented a new problem. Madeline, after the three-week hiatus from her side, noticed immediately that something was terribly wrong with her baby girl. Moskowitz confirmed her worst fears. He told the family that Debbie was severely disabled, mentally retarded, and deaf, and would require constant care to meet her basic needs, including feeding and hygiene; she would probably struggle to walk, and although difficult to predict, would never talk.

Frank and Madeline were emotionally, physically, and psychologically devastated. They already had one chronically ill child; another was unimaginable. On the surface, they had everything—love, privilege, affluence, two children—but their experience was one of uncertainty, grief, and sadness; one child with an undiagnosed, life-threatening immunological disorder, the second severely disabled. What had gone wrong?

Frank and Madeline struggled. They had another very difficult decision to make—could they, and should they, keep Debbie at home? Already, they struggled to provide Mark with the care he needed; would they have the bandwidth to ensure that Debbie received the attention and love that she needed? With aching hearts, they made the difficult decision to place Debbie in a residential home for the severely compromised. There, she would receive dignified and respectful care, of that they were certain; and they, in turn, could focus on Mark.

On the evening they drove Debbie to her new home outside of Philadelphia, they returned to their eastside apartment, weeping and speaking little; they were emotionally drained and filled with sadness. After putting their son to bed, Frank and Madeline retired to the den, shared a glass of 10-year-old Dewar's scotch, and sat on the sofa holding hands. Turning to his wife, Frank said, "I hope we made the right decision."

He retrieved from the desk drawer a handwritten note he had penned to Madeline as they prepared to take their marriage vows:

The challenges to both of us lie ahead. If there are setbacks . . . we must call on our most tremendous source of strength, our enduring love for each other.

How had he known?

How Had He Known?

Debbie's absence tormented the Niemans. They cried every day for what felt like an eternity. Mark, Madeline, and Frank were heartbroken and devastated with one-quarter of their family missing in Pennsylvania. Had they made the right decision? Perhaps it was possible for them to care for Debbie at home; perhaps they should leave the city, move to Scarsdale, Tenafly, or Greenwich; perhaps Debbie could have her own wing in a house with caregivers around the clock. She could isolate from Mark if need be. They would all be together—the entire family. Could Debbie ever forgive them? Would she ever know her parents, would she know her big brother? Frank and Madeline were guilt-ridden and beleaguered; they could not sleep, they could not eat; Frank was unable to work, they existed in a state of denial and confusion.

It took Mark to awaken them and bring the whole family back to reality. Again, he became sick—really sick—with a high fever, a cough, and shortness of breath. Madeline called Irwin Moskowitz, and he instructed her to go to the emergency room immediately. After a rapid evaluation, Mark was admitted directly to the intensive care unit. He was having difficulty breathing, his blood counts were low, and he was vulnerable to an opportunistic infection. His lung and liver function deteriorated, and his chest x-rays showed defined, discrete "cannon-ball lesions" compatible with a fungal infection—likely Aspergillus or Candida, both difficult to treat with recognized morbidity and mortality.

Madeline and Frank were terrified, their eyes and countenance betrayed their central question: was it possible to lose two children in just one month? Madeline and Frank never left Mark's side. They talked to him, encouraged him, and massaged his back and legs. "Come on, Mark, you can beat this! Please, Mark, please," they pleaded.

Broad-spectrum antibiotics and amphotericin, a new antifungal medication, were started, and oxygen was administered. The hospitalization was a long, hard slog through the mud, with slow, tedious progress. Dr. Siegal, the immunologist, suggested an experimental, yet-unproven therapy: an empiric infusion of serum immune gamma globulin. Not certain of its efficacy or contribution, it seemed to contribute and helped Mark fight the fungal infection. After two months in the hospital, he recovered, the Niemans retreated to their apartment, and Frank returned to work on 47th Street.

One evening, after reading Mark his bedtime story and tucking him into bed with a kiss on the cheek, Frank and Madeline retired to the den. Frank poured two glasses of sherry, and together they reclined on the sofa, peering out the window at the Empire State Building bathed in red, white, and blue. Reaching into his pocket, Frank pulled out a small felt box and placed it on the coffee table.

"Honey," he said, "I love you. You've been through more than anyone should ever have to go through, and I want you to have something special."

Opening the box, he presented Madeline with a flawless 5-carat, pear-shaped yellow diamond ring—a symbol of their love, their commitment, and their resilience. He recalled the handwritten note he had penned to Madeline before their wedding day and said, "We'll get through this; Mark will get through this; our love and our family will endure and be our strength."

They embraced, refilled their glasses, and cuddled together on the sofa, talking well past midnight. That night, they recommitted themselves to

Mark, promising to find the answer to his medical problems and to dedicate their lives to ensuring he got the care he needed.

The first step was to consult with medical experts. Madeline consulted Moskowitz, who in turn suggested that she consult Frank Siegel, Jerry Tannenbaum, and David Davidson, the previous chair of the department of pediatrics at Mt. Sinai and an infectious disease expert. It became apparent that the field of immunology was a nascent specialty with very few experts. The presumptive diagnosis of an immunological disorder was primarily descriptive in nature, therapies consisted of antibiotics to treat recurrent infections, and sadly, most children died. The Niemans were not deterred.

Siegel suggested two doctors, Jordan Nathan in Boston and Jay Krieger at the University of Alabama in Birmingham. Madeline contacted them and made appointments for consultations. They both wanted to review Mark's medical history prior to the visit and asked that the records be mailed to them. Moskowitz directed Madeline to the medical record department in the basement of the Klingenstein Pavilion. The clerk instructed her to complete a form in order to comply with her request to duplicate Mark's chart. "How long will this take?" Madeline asked. "When I can I pick them up?"

"I'll have them ready as soon as possible. Give me a week."

Mark's file was huge. It contained every note from every hospital admission written by Dr. Moskowitz; every note written by the interns, residents, and medical students; every consult note; every nurse note; page after page of vital signs, medications, lab results, and diagnostic x-rays. The entirety was voluminous—eight inches thick, five pounds. When Madeline returned to the record department to retrieve the copied charts, she could not believe the size of Mark's records; a quick perusal informed that much of the chart was illegible, either because the copy was of poor quality or the handwritten script entries could not be understood. Similarly, she reasoned that Drs. Nathan and Krieger had little interest in the hundreds of pages that chronicled numerical data. That night after dinner, with Mark safely in bed, Madeline and Frank each carried a complete record and placed them on the dining room table, they began the task of trying to make sense of the records.

The dining room, adjacent to the living room, was stylish and elegant, with a large mahogany art deco table situated in the middle of the room and flanked by eight high-back chairs. Beneath the table was a beautiful earth tone custom rug from Stark Carpets; the opposite walls were adorned with a wall-mounted three-door server on one and an armoire on the other.

Hunkered at the dining room table, the Niemans got to work. They decided that both records should be identical. The important information was contained in the admission note and discharge summary that was often dictated by an attending physician and typed by the hospital transcription service, thus readable. Each admission, separated from the others by dividers, also had a medication and laboratory summary page and would be included, as would all of the reports of relevant diagnostic tests and x-rays. It took them several hours to compile the two identical records of Mark's chart, which Frank then placed in sturdy envelopes. He addressed one to Dr. Nathan at Boston Children's Hospital and the other to Dr. Jay Krieger in Alabama. Madeline planned to bring the envelopes to the post office on East 70th Street in the morning. Their work done for the night, they went to sleep.

The four-hour travel time to Boston from New York is a straight ride— U.S. Route 95 the entire trip— not scenic, but direct. The Niemans arrived for their afternoon appointment with Dr. Nathan promptly at 2 p.m. They entered the lobby of the famed Boston Children's Hospital on Longwood Avenue and followed the signs to Allergy and Immunology.

Nathan, an affable man, greeted Mark and the Niemans warmly. "Good afternoon, young man, it's a pleasure to meet you."

Mark, now a precocious five-year-old, extended his right hand. "Hi, Dr. Nathan!"

Dr. Nathan told the Niemans that he had reviewed Mark's chart and thanked Frank and Madeline for summarizing and distilling it to a manageable size. "So, Mark, here is what I would like to do today. I'll talk to your mom and dad first, then examine you and have some blood drawn, and then we'll all talk again. Is that okay with you?"

Mark nodded. "Sure."

After speaking with the Niemans and examining Mark, Dr. Nathan explained that the field of immunology was relatively new and descriptive in nature, but that there were new discoveries made regularly. He concluded that, based on the early onset of Mark's infections and their frequency, Mark had a congenital immunodeficiency disorder, though the precise defect or abnormality was unknown. He told them it was interesting that when Mark became ill, his blood counts dropped, which exacerbated the infection and made it more difficult to treat. He was unable to determine if the low counts precipitated the infection or were a result of the infection. He suggested routine surveillance blood counts on a regular time interval, perhaps every two weeks for a few months to elucidate the answer. He showed the Niemans a paper he had co-authored with his colleague, Oscar Charles, regarding the administration of gamma globulin therapy for patients with primary immunodeficiency diseases, and believed infusions of intravenous hyper-immune globulin would be worth a try to determine if it might ameliorate Mark's infections.

Satisfied and hopeful, the family bade goodbye to Dr. Nathan.

"Thanks, Dr. Nathan," Mark said.

"My pleasure, young man. I would like to see you again next year; would that be all right with you?"

"Sure."

That evening, the Niemans went to Faneuil Hall, had clam chowder and fried lobster for dinner at Legal Seafood, and returned to the Copley Square

Hotel for the night. They tried their best to make the trip an adventure and even began to allow themselves to feel hopeful.

However, barely back in New York City, Mark soon became ill again with high fever, low blood counts, shortness of breath, and pneumonia. He and Madeline spent the next 18 days on Falk 3 at Mt. Sinai. He received a gamma globulin infusion, routine by now, which seemed to help.

Jay Krieger at the University of Alabama became a friend and confidant of Frank and Madeline. He spoke with Jordan Nathan, and they also asked Elizabeth Bussell at Memorial Sloan Kettering in New York to join their brain trust. Collectively, they suggested that Mark receive prophylactic monthly gamma globulin infusions, regardless of his own endogenous production, to keep his levels elevated. They also suggested pursuing a bone marrow transplant—a new experimental therapy primarily used as a treatment modality for refractory leukemia and lymphoma, which had recently been attempted in a child with a congenital immunological disorder. There were only a few institutions and physician scientists that performed transplants: Donnall Thomas, University of Washington, George Santos at Johns Hopkins, and Robert Good at the University of Minnesota. Hypothetically, it should work to replace Mark's immune system with a new stronger, healthier infection-fighting structure. The caveat—there existed only one potential donor: Debbie. An allogeneic bone marrow transplant could only be performed using marrow from a matched sibling, and the possibility of a match between Debbie and Mark was one in four.

The prospect of using Debbie as a bone marrow donor terrified Madeline and Frank. There were ethical issues to consider. In addition, if she were a match, the transplant successful, and Mark survived, would her bad genes, those that caused severe retardation, become part of Mark's DNA? No one could answer the question. Nevertheless, a decision was made to determine if Mark and Debbie were a match. Blood was drawn for HLA typing and mixed lymphocyte cultures (MLCs) on both children and sent to Baltimore, the Santos lab at Hopkins. Unfortunately—or fortunately, depending on one's perspective—they did not match and the MLCs revealed a non-compatible result. Decision averted.

The Niemans enrolled Mark in Birch Wathen, a small co-ed school on East 77th Street, the same school Madeline had attended two decades prior. The school environment was perfect for Mark, and he made friends easily, enjoying his classes and showing an interest in squash and tennis.

Madeline and Frank were determined to allow Mark's life be as normal as possible. When he was well, he had good energy and enjoyed travelling to new places. The Niemans visited Scottsdale, Arizona, the Beverly Hills Hotel and Disneyland in Los Angeles, and grandparents in Boca Raton. Looking for a second home, they investigated Connecticut rather than the Hamptons, where they would have an easier route back into the city, should they need to return to the hospital in an emergency. The towns they visited were serviced by Metro North and would allow Frank to easily commute to work in the city during the week.

They settled on a modest, contemporary home on a tree-lined street within walking distance of town, the village park, a public beach, tennis courts, and a golf club. It was perfectly situated on half an acre, with an open floor plan, a large family room with a wonderful fireplace hearth, four bedrooms, a sunroom, and a porch. There was also a fenced-in yard with a swing set and jungle gym. The entire family, but especially Mark, adored the house and Connecticut.

Life continued as normal, with Mark continuing to periodically become ill. It was the same ordeal every time, with fever, pneumonia, and low blood counts, but the gamma globulin infusions made a distinct difference, helping Mark to recover more rapidly with shorter hospitalizations.

One summer, Frank bought a 31-foot sailboat, which he named the 'MAN' for Mark Alan Nieman. The boat, harbored in the town marina, permitted easy access to the Long Island Sound and east coast ports. Captain Mark loved to sail. The family ventured to Newport, Martha's Vineyard, Nantucket, and Cape Cod where they would dock at night and sleep on the boat. They all enjoyed sailing, especially Mark, who soon became quite capable at the helm.

As Mark grew older, his early teenage years were difficult. His frequent hospitalizations made him different at a time when he simply wanted to fit in, and although he remained well between hospitalizations, he knew that he was not like other kids. All Mark wanted was to be with his friends, playing tennis or baseball, or sailing, but Frank and Madeline were compelled to protect him and keep him sheltered, away from crowds. They were understandably protective, afraid to expose him to anyone who had even the slightest cold. He tried desperately to be upbeat, but he was frustrated.

One evening, he said to his parents, "I wish I had leukemia—at least then the doctors could treat me. I'd get chemotherapy and I'd be fine, cured. Mom, Dad, you're both smart—please do something. I've had enough; I don't want to do this anymore."

One afternoon, Carrie French paged me.

"Yes, Carrie?"

Larry Schultz had called; he said Mark Nieman had been admitted and his white count is 300,000.

"I'll be right there—Falk 3? I'll meet you at the nurse's station."

Carrie French was terrific. A graduate of University of Pennsylvania and the Mt. Sinai School of Medicine, she chose to take one year in clinical hematology and oncology before entering general pediatrics in Westchester County, north of the city; however, her real claim to fame was that she was an Olympic-level figure skater. She had skated with and competed against Dorothy Hamill, the woman's gold medal winner at the 1976 Innsbruck, Austria Winter Games. Carrie, 10 years removed from international competition, remained a beautiful, graceful skater; she enjoyed skating with my daughter, Lauren, and whenever she had time, taught her twists and twirls on the Wollman Rink ice in Central Park.

Carrie was waiting for me with slide in hand. As we walked to our office on the fourth floor of the service building, she said that Mark had a massively

enlarged liver and spleen. We postulated that his illness had finally declared itself—leukemia. We entered the laboratory and sat at the four-head
teaching microscope. After placing the slide on the stage and applying oil
for 100x magnification, we viewed cells the likes of which I had never seen
before. My partner, Mitchell Moche, joined us and was similarly amazed.

Mitchell Moche is one of the best people I know. Really smart and well-
trained at Albert Einstein College of Medicine and the Children's Hospital of Philadelphia, he is honest and hardworking. We made an excellent
team, though we were different in so many ways; we complimented one
another. Physically, we were opposites, I was 5-foot 9, he 6-foot 5; I was
glib, excitable, and he was reserved, calm; I enjoyed sports, while he was
studious, preferred reading books, and going on walks with his wife, Eleanor. I practiced my Jewish faith and religion twice a year in the fall at
the High Holidays; Mitchell was Orthodox, connected to his synagogue
in Englewood, and practiced his faith every day of every month of every
year. My wife Alicia and I enjoyed traveling to faraway places and exploring
different cultures; Mitchell and Eleanor only went to Israel. Yet, when it
came to patients and our responsibilities at Mt. Sinai, we were on the same
page—a well-oiled machine, a Swiss watch, a Japanese bullet train.

We agreed that these were not lymphoblasts or myeloblasts. Morphologically,
we were dumbfounded; we could not assign lineage to the cells. They were
large and the nuclear chromatin was homogeneous, with nucleoli and abundant basophilic cytoplasm. They were abnormal; of that there was no doubt,
but beyond that, we were clueless. We postulated that perhaps they could
be mesenchymal, histiocytic, or dendritic in origin. Mitchell, Carrie, and I
concluded that a bone marrow examination would not enhance our ability
to make a diagnosis. The white blood cell count had risen to 400,000. His-
tochemical stains, sheep-red blood cell rosettes, and surface immunoglobulin
could be assessed using a sample of the peripheral blood. Mitchell thought
it was a good idea to show the slides to Janice Klopkin, head of the adult
leukemia service, as Carrie and I went back to Falk 3 to update the Niemans.

"Can we talk here, including Mark, or would you prefer to have privacy?"
I asked.

"Here is fine."

"Well, where to begin?"

"Michael, Carrie, we know something is going on. This is not typical Mark. Tell us what you think, be honest."

"It appears as though Mark has some kind of leukemia. We're not certain what type, but frankly we cannot imagine anything else. He has a large liver and spleen, and his white count is over 400,000. Mitchell Moche is bringing slides and peripheral blood to the hemepath lab for additional testing so hopefully we will have an answer soon."

Frank, Madeline, and Mark were confused. They didn't know how to react or respond. A leukemia diagnosis terrified them, yet it represented something concrete, something that we would be able to treat. Frank asked, "Can we send the slides and material to Drs. Nathan and Krieger for their opinion? George Eisman is a friend of ours, can you let him know also?"

"Of course."

Some things didn't jive. Despite the white count being off the charts elevated, Mark was not otherwise sick. In fact, he felt well, with no fever and no evidence of infection or pneumonia. He was not anemic, and his platelet count was normal. In most instances, when leukemia is diagnosed, the red cell and platelet cell lines are affected, but that was not the case with Mark. The hemepath lab was unable to establish lineage, and they thought the blast cells, if one could even refer to them as blasts, were of histiocytic origin. Janice Klopkin was at a loss to help; review of the case by Nathan and Krieger and their colleagues in Alabama and Boston was indeterminate as well. We were perplexed as to the diagnosis and how best to treat Mark, or, better stated, *whether* to treat Mark.

We waited.

Our small team gathered on Friday morning in Moche's corner office, seated around his enormous desk, for our weekly LTA—"let's talk about"—conference. Boruch Levine, our children's radiotherapist, and Steve Bleicher, our pediatric surgeon, joined as well. We ordered lunch from Pete's Luncheonette; I had my usual BLT; Mitchell, a tuna fish sandwich; Carrie, Karen, and Betty, our two nurses, and June Schwartz, the social worker, had salads. We discussed Mark first. We needed a plan, recognizing that at times, the best decision is no decision. "Do no harm."

Mitchell pointed out that the peripheral blood count of 400,000 had risk of thrombosis. He thought we should try to lower the count slowly, over the course of a few days—a good point. We discussed leukapheresis as a possibility, but decided on using cyclophosphamide, a chemotherapy drug, and prednisone. I discussed our recommendations with Frank and Madeline, and they agreed with the plan; they understood our concerns about the high count, and were in favor of proceeding slowly, cautiously. Mark was different, unique. We administered the Cytoxan and began a five-day course of steroids. The next morning, Mark's white blood cell count was 50 percent reduced; two days later he was out of bed and walking the halls, smiling and feeling great. By the fifth day, his last on prednisone, the count was under 25,000, and he was discharged home. We never did understand what transpired or what the identity of those bizarre cells might be, but it mattered little, Mark was well, until the presumed next time.

I, not infrequently, tell my young colleagues, "In medicine, things happen that we don't understand with no apparent explanation, but the important message is to live with it and accept it as long as your patient gets better."

To celebrate, Frank and Madeline asked Mark if he would enjoy a trip. "Where would you like to visit?"

"How about Europe? I've never been. Can we go to London and Paris? We've been studying European history in school!"

Two days later, the Nieman family left for London and Paris. They had a terrific time sightseeing, visiting Buckingham Palace, Big Ben, and museums, and shopping at Harrods. In Paris, they visited the Eiffel Tower, saw the Mona Lisa at the Louvre, and walked along Les Champs-Élysées. They loved Paris, especially at night—"The City of Lights." The night before they would return home, Frank told Madeline and Mark that he had a special surprise.

"We have one more place to visit before New York. I thought you would enjoy a few days at the beach in Capri."

Madeline just smiled, overjoyed to see Mark so happy.

After their European vacation, Mark returned to Birch Wathen, and was thrilled to return to his friends and classmates. As an introduction to the eighth grade, the school planned an overnight whale watching trip to Cape Cod. Madeline was reluctant to allow him to go in such close quarters with other kids, and in the cold and damp September water. She could conjure up a multitude of reasons to say no, but she didn't; reluctantly, she agreed. Mark had returned home from his stay in the hospital and subsequent trip to Europe emboldened, fearless, and strong. He felt invincible.

One Saturday in early October, the Niemans drove to Princeton University; Frank's alma mater, the Columbia University Lions were to do battle with the Princeton Tigers on the Palmer Stadium gridiron. Located in central New Jersey, Princeton is about an hour and a half drive south of the city. The university and town is idyllic—the university, with its collegiate gothic style architecture, and the town, packed with quaint stores and restaurants, its architecture dating back to the Revolutionary War.

The village was packed with people, most dressed in orange and black, Princeton's colors, though Frank and Mark wore Columbia blue sweatshirts and hats. They ate breakfast—banana pancakes, Mark's favorite—at the PJ's Pancake House on Nassau Street, right in the center of town, just a couple blocks from Nassau Hall. Before the game, Frank and Mark were on the field tossing a football and mingling with the players on the Columbia team sideline during their warm-ups. All in all, it was an awesome experience made that much better by the final score: Columbia, 27–Princeton, 18.

Mark was on a roll. He looked and felt better than any time in recent memory. He had become Mr. Full Steam Ahead. He was enjoying school, spending time with his friends, playing tennis, and sailing on the weekends. He even became a quasi-DJ, "The MAN (Mark Alan Nieman) Session," spinning Motown, of course.

The evening after the football game, with Mark fast asleep in bed, Frank and Madeline enjoyed a quiet moment in the den. They shared a glass of Harvey's and watched Cher and Nicholas Cage in *Moonstruck*.

Frank allowed himself to dream aloud. "Could it be true—could Mark be well? Is it conceivable that he is outgrowing the cycle of infection and illness? Is puberty changing his body, strengthening his immune system?"

"Honey, don't. Let's just try to enjoy him while we can. I cannot think in 'what ifs'. Just watch the movie."

Madeline's restraint proved to be rational. Before long, Mark developed a cough—a non-stop, hacking cough, accompanied by a high fever. He sensed something was different this time. Now 15 years old, he was frightened.

"Mom, Dad," he implored. "Do something!"

Mark was admitted directly from the emergency room to the intensive care unit. His blood counts were normal, liver normal, but his oxygen saturation was in the low 80s. Moskowitz and Elizabeth Bussell, who left Sloan Kettering and now worked at Mt. Sinai, ordered an immediate infusion of intravenous gamma globulin. A chest x-ray revealed diffuse, patchy infiltrates bilaterally—both lungs were involved. Mitchell Moche and I went to the ICU to offer our assistance, anything to help. Dick Poller, Chief of Pulmonology, Alec Black, and Bob Davidson, David's son, from Infectious Disease, were also in the unit. Could this be pneumocystis carinii?

"Do we need a lung biopsy? Dick, what do you think?"

Mitchell mentioned that there was a new drug available, Pentamidine, specifically for P. carinii that Phil Pizzo at the NIH and Walter Hughes at St. Jude's recently reported had had miraculous results. Mitchell offered to make a few calls.

Dick and Alec told the Niemans that a bronchoscopy to confirm a diagnosis would be helpful. He told them that Mark would need anesthesia to do the procedure and would need to be intubated to help deliver oxygen to his heart, brain, lungs, and other vital organs.

Terrified and crying, Mark realized this moment, this very moment, could be the last moment that he could see his parents, talk to his parents, hold his mother's hand.

Again, he begged them, "Mom, Dad, do something!"

When the procedure, performed at the bedside, had been completed, Mark seemed comfortable and stable while intubated on a respirator. Mitchell spoke directly to Pizzo who offered to release Pentamidine, but it would take several days to get to New York. Madeline had a solution: "I'll go to Washington tomorrow and pick it up."

Madeline took a cab from Mt. Sinai to LaGuardia, purchased a ticket on the Delta Airlines shuttle, and arrived at National Airport in D.C. From there, she traveled to the sprawling National Institute of Health campus in Bethesda, Maryland, and located Building 10. She asked the cab to wait and took the elevator to Pizzo's office on the eighth floor. The Pentamidine was packed and on the desk in the waiting room. The doctor heard Madeline thanking his assistant and came out of his office. "Good luck, Mrs. Nieman. I hope this helps your son."

Retracing her steps, Madeline immediately returned to National Airport and caught the next shuttle back to LaGuardia. She went from New York to Washington and back in less than five hours. But for Mark, five hours was an eternity, as his condition worsened and the chest x- ray revealed a virtual "white-out." His fever was 104; his oxygen saturation in the low 90s; carbon dioxide at 52 percent, markedly elevated; all ominous indicators.

The Pentamidine was administered, but would it be too late to save his life? Mark's plea, "Do something, do something," reverberated over and over in Madeline's head, but there was nothing to do but wait and hope the new medication would help and that it wasn't too late.

Frank and Madeline were numb, speechless, mute, in total disbelief. They had done everything humanly possible for Mark, including the decision a decade ago to institutionalize Debbie to preserve and prolong his life. They were tormented. They consulted the best doctors, protected him, yet still he was sick. They were all about Mark, every minute of every day, and now he was about to slip away

Mark became edematous. He experienced multiple organ failure, and the Pentamidine did little to reverse his rapid demise. Developments happened precipitously, within hours. Word spread quickly through the hospital: "Mark Nieman is dying."

Mitchell Moche, Carrie French, Larry Schultz, Dick Poller, Irwin Moskowitz, Elizabeth Bussell, Alec Black, the nurses and staff, and I congregated in the ICU. Frank and Madeline had become like family to us. Madeline noted a single tear on Mark's left cheek, just one symbolic tear.

And then he was gone.

We were all in shock. No one could speak. Frank and Madeline robotically thanked us all for everything we had done for Mark, gathered their belongings, and left the ICU. Holding hands wordlessly, they walked for hours— down Fifth Avenue to Central Park West, to Madison Avenue and down to Gramercy Park, up Third Avenue to their apartment. Frank collapsed on the sofa in the den, while Madeline retired to their bedroom; they both needed to be alone with their thoughts and grief.

Mark's words echo in Madeline's head: *Do something . . .*

Do Something!

Eight hundred twenty-one physician scientists; 28 post-doctoral fellow-ships; 4 endowed chairs for pediatric immunology research; 150 programs at 379 centers in 294 cities representing 86 countries located on 6 continents; this is the story of how Frank and Madeline Nieman did something.

Mark's funeral was at the Frank Campbell Funeral Home on Madison Avenue. The mourners—family, Mark's friends from school and camp, Frank and Madeline's friends and business associates, hospital friends, doctors, nurses, and staff—filled the sanctuary, overflowing onto the Avenue. Frank and Madeline attempted to be polite, accepting condolences from hundreds of people, but it was impossible. They were unable to speak; they could not utter Mark's name; there was no solace to comfort them, their loss too great. No more sailing, tennis, playing ball in the park; no more Columbia football games; no more travel to California or Florida; no more trips to Europe or the African safari to Botswana and Kenya they'd planned. Their beloved son was now just a memory.

The Niemans desperately wanted to be alone with their own thoughts. The *shiva* at their apartment was a necessity, but it was painful. The platters of food from Zabars, bagels and smoked fish, cold cut meats for sandwiches, and pastries were wasted. No one could eat. The Niemans' little family of four was now two—Debbie, poor Debbie, in her own world in Pennsylvania, had no idea that she had even had a brother. For Frank and Madeline, who had dedicated their existence to their son's illness, it was impossible to fill the void. They were isolated, unsure, and alone. They wandered around blankly, pausing to pick up family photos, then setting them down and walking away.

Frank was unable to work. He tried his best to piece together the information surrounding Marks's illness. He pored over medical records from Mark's many hospitalizations, consults, and conversations with experts. The Niemans knew the story of the *The Boy in the Plastic Bubble*, popularized by the movie starring John Travolta—was that similar to Mark's plight? They questioned whether their son should have been rigidly isolated but unequivocally decided that their decision had been the right one for Mark; although his life was short, he had lived it to the fullest. Frank and Madeline did an exhaustive search regarding immunodeficiency. They were not doctors, but they were intelligent, asking questions and absorbing everything they learned. They questioned the basic concepts—what is the immune system, how does it operate, what are its components? They concluded that there was very little information about children with defects and dysfunction of the immune system. Medical science and advancement had progressed significantly more diagnostically and therapeutically for childhood cancer and heart disease; it became apparent that the number of children afflicted by immune disorders was not known, nor were the signs and symptoms of the disease.

Madeline and Frank recognized that they could no longer do something for Mark, but they *could* do something for other children like him.

They spoke to Elizabeth Bussell, Jay Krieger, Jordan Nathan, and Robert Good at Memorial Sloan Kettering to solicit ideas. Though all four were revered, respected physician scientists, their perspectives were disappointingly narrow and self-serving. Independently, they tried to convince the Niemans to support their research enterprise, but Frank and Madeline wanted more; they wanted answers to their questions. *What exactly is an immunodeficiency disease? What are the signs and symptoms of immune disorders? Can these diseases be prevented?* Their goal was to fundamentally change the landscape, plant seeds, and watch them grow and flourish. Their goal was to create a different world for patients.

Elizabeth Bussell had an idea. She suggested to the Niemans that they sponsor an international conference. They would be able to bring the best scientists and medical minds together to establish a world renowned, international conference of the leading immunologists. They asked Elizabeth if this was even possible. Had such a conference been done before? How much would it cost? Where to begin?

Frank and Madeline discussed the idea with friends and family. They felt they had no choice but to try to make a difference—to *do something*. They committed themselves fully to the project, totally immersing themselves in the health and well-being of their new offspring, their third child: The Mark Nieman Foundation. They created an independent 501(c)(3) charity, formed an advisory board of directors, and set out to educate the world about immunological disorders and to create a better world for patients and families. The foundation was created to celebrate Mark's life; a tribute to his optimism and courage, not in memory of his death. Its mission was clear—discover, educate, support, advocate.

Madeline's cousin offered the first donation to the MAN Foundation, $500. They were on their way, full steam ahead, just like Mark. Frank sold his jewelry and diamond business to devote all of his time, energy, and resources to the foundation, but they needed money. Madeline proved to be an extraordinary fundraiser. She was connected, with a wide circle of family, friends, and acquaintances, and she did not hesitate to reach out and ask them all to help save the lives of children. She spoke with leadership of pharmaceutical and biotech companies, asking for their assistance in defining and developing immunological innovation platforms and sponsorship money to advance and promote the ideals of the foundation.

Frank and Madeline hosted annual galas at The Plaza, Waldorf, or Museum of Natural History with over 1,000 guests. The dinners were a highlight of the New York social calendar and raised millions of dollars.

The medical advisory board, led by Drs. Bussell, Nathan Good, and Krieger, worked with the American Red Cross and the Centers for Disease Control to formulate 10 signs and symptoms of immune disorders, including frequent infections of the ears, sinuses, pneumonia, skin abscesses, and sepsis that did not respond to antibiotics. These warning signs of primary immunodeficiency have since been translated into 50 languages.

The Mark Nieman Foundation has organized more than 50 international scientific symposia, including global meetings in collaboration with the World Health Organization and International Union of Immunological Societies in Europe, Asia, and the Americas. The Foundation has collaborated with the National Institutes of Health, the Centers for Disease Control, and the public and private sector to conduct a public awareness, physician education, and public service campaigns that has resulted in an ever-increasing number of patients identified, referred, diagnosed, treated, and saved.

Frank and Madeline appeared before the United States Congress to garner the support of Senators Joe Lieberman and Al D'Amato, from Connecticut and New York respectively, to advocate for newborn screening for severe combined immunodeficiency disorders (SCID), and in 2010 convinced Kathleen Sebelius, Secretary of Health and Human Services in the Obama administration, to recommend SCID to the National Core Panel, where it would be added as part of the hereditary disease assessment panel at birth. Hundreds of infants have been diagnosed and have received life-saving stem cell transplants secondary to this initiative.

The Mark Nieman Foundation, by supporting scientific forums, research funding, and advocacy, has been a critical catalyst for the increased pace of scientific discovery and positive change for health policy around the world.

In 2007, the foundation celebrated a monumental achievement, the creation of the Mark Nieman Immunology Research Building at the Harvard University School of Medicine. The work of the MAN Foundation continues to this day. The vital research and dissemination of knowledge supported by the philanthropy of Frank and Madeline is beyond comprehension. An incredible transformation founded in sadness and despair has positively affected thousands of lives, one at a time.

"Mark, we did something."

HANK HELD

Call A Rapid

My routine is to arrive at 8 to review the patient notes and the results of the morning labs in order to familiarize myself with potential problems. We then convene in the team room, a room without windows that was tired and worn the day the Morgan Stanley Children's Hospital opened 15 years ago. Along the far wall are three computers and a printer. The table in the center of the room is always a disaster area—papers strewn about, last night's pizza, and three-day old tasteless kosher cookies that, frankly, were not worth eating even when fresh. The mess used to bother me and I would often spend 10 minutes every morning tossing the garbage out and cleaning the table and work area, but not any longer; it just didn't seem to be important in the scheme of things, and no one else seemed to care, so why should I?

My team that morning consisted of two first-year residents, Katie Greene and Amanda Sanchez. Charlie Bradley one of the first-year hematology-oncology fellows, and hopefully Lisa Jones, the leukemia-lymphoma clinical nurse practitioner, would join as well. The residents were usually really smart, well educated, and hard working. Katie and Amanda certainly fit this profile. Katie graduated from Princeton and Duke University Medical School, and Amanda went to Columbia University for undergrad and the Vagelos College of Physicians and Surgeons of Columbia University for medical school—both impressive, but so young. There were times when I felt intellectually inferior to these young physicians-in-training. My education, in comparison, was very pedestrian: Dickinson College in Carlisle, Pennsylvania and Upstate Medical Center in Syracuse, New York. I went to Dickinson because I wanted to play basketball and I thought I would be able to do so at a small Division 3 college. I chose Upstate rather than New York University or the Albany College of Medicine, both private medical schools, because being a New York State resident I had a Regents Scholarship to a state school, thus the cost of my medical education was under a $1,000 per year, no loans needed. Nevertheless, after 40 years as a pediatric oncologist I still seem to get the job done efficiently and effectively.

"Good morning all, should we sit or walk?"

"Let's walk."

We collected our papers, pens, clipboards, and patient lists, left the team room, and assembled in the Pod 1 nursing station. Amanda unplugged the cow, our portable computer, and Charlie grabbed the visual interpreter computer device, an invaluable piece of technology that allows us to communicate with our non-English speaking patients. I had hoped that one of the residents was fluent in Spanish, but Amanda, although of Puerto Rican heritage, spoke only English with her family.

There were 14 inpatients on the service: two in the pediatric intensive care unit on the 11th floor, and 12 on Tower 5, the oncology floor. Of the 12, six were Spanish speaking, one Arabic, one Chinese, and one Russian. The diversity of our patient population was one of the great strengths of the program. We were a community hospital for the Dominican population in Washington Heights as well as a referral hospital, for not only the New York metropolitan area, but for patients around the world. We'd make good use of the mobile translator today.

As a group, we moved towards Room 501.

"Did someone call his nurse?" Lisa Jones asked.

"We did, but Valerie isn't available; she is too busy with another patient."

Before we entered the room or discussed the case, we tried to engage the nurse caring for each child at the bedside. Sometimes they are able to add insight that we might otherwise not appreciate, though they are hardly ever able to join rounds. There is no doubt that they are busy, as the bedside care of children with cancer is hard and demanding work, but one needs to know whether they are too busy because the floor nurses are short-staffed and overwhelmed, or whether joining rounds is not a priority.

Standing outside the room, Amanda began to present the case to the team.

"Hank is our three-year-old male with acute lymphoblastic leukemia."

"Amanda, forgive me," I said, "but he is a three-year-old with ALL. If he belongs to anyone, it is to his parents."

"Sorry, you're right."

I told the group that Hank was a fascinating case. He had presented with headaches and an unsteady gait. His mother, Heather Held, was a physician. She graduated from the College of Physicians and Surgeons of Columbia University, completed her residency at Yale, and had just started a fertility fellowship at Mt. Sinai Hospital when she noticed that Hank was having difficulty walking. Sensing that something was wrong, she made arrangements for him to have an MRI, which revealed a brain tumor.

Hank was evaluated by Max Granstein, Chief of Pediatric Neurosurgery, who performed a craniotomy to remove the tumor. Surgery went extremely well, and Hank had a short post-operative course without incident, followed by a rapid recovery.

The pathology was consistent with a low-grade pilocytic astrocytoma, a slow-growing malignant tumor. When completely removed surgically, no further treatment is needed, and the cure rate is very high, approaching 100 percent. However, when the neuropathologist reviewed the tumor sample, he found abnormal lymphocytes in the margins of tumor that were consistent with lymphoblasts.

Prior to surgery, Hank had done no blood work, not even a complete blood count. Granstein's routine, in an otherwise healthy child, is not to perform blood work before surgery. Given the pathology findings, however, we obtained a CBC and a peripheral blood-flow cytometry, which is used to find abnormal leukemia populations in the blood. Both revealed abnormal results: white count of 15,700 x 10³ /mL, Hgb 7.2 g/dL, and a platelet count of 68,000 x 10³ /mL; the differential had 47 percent lymphocytes and 24 percent atypical lymphoblasts; the flow cytometry was also positive for leukemia. To be perfectly candid, he was fortunate to have had a major brain operation without incident and no excessive bleeding.

To confirm a diagnosis of leukemia, a bone marrow aspirate, biopsy, and a lumbar puncture with intrathecal cytarabine were performed. Our suspicions were verified—Hank had B-cell acute lymphoblastic leukemia, ALL. Dr. Pace and her husband, Max Held, were in disbelief. Within one week, their beautiful son had been diagnosed with not one, but two simultaneous cancers.

The low-grade pilocytic astrocytoma had probably been in the posterior part of his brain near the cerebellum for months, perhaps longer, but when totally resected they usually do not need any additional therapy, just observation, close monitoring. Our concerns and efforts needed to be focused on treating and curing the leukemia.

Lisa Jones, the leukemia nurse practitioner, is incredibly knowledgeable about the basic principles of ALL. She is a tall, thin, marathon-running fool with two passions: caring for children with leukemia and running. Her goal was to run all of the major marathons worldwide. She has already completed New York, Chicago, Tokyo, and Boston. I like Lisa; she does a great job.

As a group, we talked about risk group stratification predicated on prognostic variables at the time of diagnosis. Low-risk patients receive standard therapy and have a cure rate of 90–95 percent, whereas high-risk patients have a poorer outlook and require more intensive chemotherapy treatment with a predicted cure rate between 70–80 percent. Hank was in the low-risk group—two years of age, low white blood cell count, pre-B phenotype, and favorable leukemic cell cytogenetics, ETV6/RUNX 1 positivity; an extremely good prognostic variable and compatible with an extremely high cure rate.

The diagnostic lumbar puncture was negative for leukemia; however, the central nervous system was violated at surgery, the cerebrospinal contaminated, thus positive, Hank would need additional lumbar punctures with intrathecal meds administered.

Historically, the recognition that leukemia cells invade the brain and the CSF, the protective fluid that surrounds the brain, was such a monumental discovery that it transformed a near-fatal illness into a practically curable, chronic illness. Drs. Hal Moore and Simon Peters made an observation in the late 1960s while working at St. Jude's Hospital in Memphis, Tennessee. They theorized that if the leukemia cells were present, they needed to be treated, and if they were not present, prophylactic therapy to prevent them from passing from the blood into the central nervous system was needed. Initially, patients received radiotherapy to the brain and the entire spinal cord as well as the instillation of chemotherapy drugs directly into the CSF, called intrathecal therapy. This treatment was very effective and increased the cure rate of children with acute lymphoblastic leukemia from 10–20 percent to greater than 50 percent. However, the therapy proved to be too toxic with too many side effects such as an increased risk of cognitive deficits, additional cancers, endocrine problems, and growth disturbances. Therefore, today, we use only intrathecal medication and use radiotherapy to the brain only if overt central nervous system disease exists.

Hank was admitted from the clinic two days prior after an anaphylactic reaction to PEG asparaginase. He previously received PEG during induction and tolerated it fine. In the next phase, consolidation, Hank received the medication again. However, as the infusion of the PEG traversed through his port-catheter tubing into his veins, he developed huge, red, blotchy hives across his entire body, an obvious allergic reaction caused by a release of histamine and inflammatory cytokines—quite dramatic. He immediately received an antihistamine, steroids, and an anti-inflammatory drug, and the reaction abated.

The DFCI protocol makes note of allergic reactions to PEG; a provision exists to re-challenge the patient and administer the drug with premeds: Benadryl, Tylenol, and methylprednisolone, a steroid. Hank's mother and father were appropriately very anxious, but agreed to a second infusion of PEG. We told Heather and Max that allergic reactions are not uncommon, and in similar patients with the premeds, it was safe to try again. PEG asparaginase, part of the backbone of the treatment protocol, is an excellent, active agent in the therapeutic armamentarium against ALL, if possible it should be continued.

Amanda continued her brief presentation Hank's vital signs were stable, afebrile, he had an excellent night—his pulse, blood pressure, and oxygen saturation were all normal. He ate breakfast, got dressed in his Ralph Lauren blue checked polo shirt and tan chinos. His parents asked if he could go home.

"Sure, let's say hello to the family and discharge him."

As we entered the room, it was apparent that everyone was ready for home. The overnight bags were packed and placed at the door, toys, and additional three-year-old paraphernalia in shopping bags ready as well.

Hank, a brown-haired, blue-eyed boy, smiled and showed me his iPad with the Paw Patrol playing. When he felt well, he was all smiles and babbling talk. He always had the obligatory miniature truck or plane in his left hand that he willingly shared with whoever engaged him. At three years old, he was too young to recognize the significance of what was happening to him and around him. Hank knew me by name: "Hi, Dr. Weiner!"

"Good morning, Hank! How are you today?"

"Good."

Hank's father asked, "What's next?"

"We'll see you in clinic next week and discuss where we go from here. We have many excellent options available, I promise. For now, no medication except the Bactrim as always; go home, do something fun, and be calm."

The prior Tuesday was a beautiful clear day as I looked out on the view from the pediatric oncology clinic on the seventh floor of the Irving Pavilion. The building and the clinical floors of the Irving Cancer Center are named after Herbert and Florence Irving, major benefactors to the entire cancer enterprise and to Columbia University Medical Center. In order to secure the gift from Herb Irving for the renovation of the pediatric oncology outpatient space, he insisted that the facility be located in the Irving Pavilion, contiguous to the adult oncology outpatient units on floors 8–14. When the space was renovated in the late 1990s it was wonderful, bright, well-conceived, and functional. Twenty years later the unit is tired, and no longer conducive to the needs of the program. In addition, it is far-removed from the Morgan Stanley Children's Hospital, which is problematic for the physicians, staff, patients, and families.

The infusion area on IP-7 is a large, open space surrounded by floor to ceiling windows on two sides. On a clear day, the view is unobstructed and spectacular. To the south, the Freedom Tower in lower Manhattan resides high above the skyline, and to the west sit the George Washington Bridge, the Hudson River Fort Lee, New Jersey, and the cliffs of the Palisades. As I gaze south, I always picture the image of the burning and falling World Trade Center Towers; the devastation and senseless loss of life on September 11, 2001 is indelibly imprinted in my mind—the image is one I will never forget.

I also remember 9-11 for another reason, as it was the first time I met the Queen family. Ten-year-old John was diagnosed with stage IV Hodgkin's lymphoma. With a backdrop of the crumbling towers, the world of the Queen family was similarly crushed as they endured their own personal tragedy. This juxtaposition remains a powerful memory.

Hank, Heather, and Max arrived at the Irving Pavilion seventh floor before 9 a.m. They registered at the front desk, and Carol Teri, the triage clinic nurse took his vital signs: temperature, height, weight, heart rate, and blood pressure, and entered the results into the computer. Hank felt comfortable on the floor, knew the routine, and walked to the infusion area in the southwest corner of the floor. He was carrying his truck in his left hand, and the iPad was tucked under his right arm. Although Heather and Max trusted me, they were tense and nervous; they accepted the collective judgment of the experts and believed what we were about to attempt was conceivable, possible, worth the attempt. PEG asparaginase is an excellent drug.

Max signed the consent document. Neither he or Heather had questions; they were prepared and the staff was prepared—all hands-on board. We were prepared to give another dosage of PEG asparaginase.

Hank settled onto his father's lap on one of the large, blue reclining chairs in the infusion area. His favorite nurse, Jessica, came by to greet the family and gave her favorite patient a hug. Jessica worked part-time in the clinic, as she was going to school to complete her degree as a nurse practitioner; however, she always checked the roster to be certain she was working when Hank and his parents were scheduled for a visit.

Using sterile technique, she carefully inserted a needle into Hank's port-a-catheter, the venous access device. Success, blood return. Jessica drew three tubes of blood for a CBC, chemical profile, and pancreatic enzymes that must be assessed prior to administering PEG asparaginase, and started an IV with normal saline. The lab values resulted quickly, excellent, all normal.

I suggested that we begin to move Hank to a bed rather than the recliner. Jessica placed the heart monitor leads on Hank's chest and put a pulse oximeter on his finger. Oxygen was ready if necessary, epinephrine, methylprednisolone were placed at the ready if needed. Hopefully all these precautions would prove to be unnecessary, but I am certain that Hank's parents appreciated the fact that we were prepared for any emergency. Hank's mom, Dr. Pace, no doubt appreciated the extra precautions.

"Did we pick up the PEG from the pharmacy?"

"Yes, it's here, and we also have all the premeds drawn up and ready to go."

Jessica gave him the Tylenol using a syringe, squirting the pink liquid into his mouth. He made a face but took the medicine like a trooper.

Jessica administered the methylprednisolone and Benadryl premeditations intravenously.

Carin Schultz, one of the senior clinic nurses that I have worked with for more than 20 years, brought the PEG asparaginase medication to the bedside. Everyone stopped what they were doing, the clinic came to a standstill; we were all apprehensive. Hank had previously had an allergic reaction to the PEG, but a full-blown anaphylactic allergic response is sudden, dramatic, terrifying, and potentially life-threatening.

Our team was experienced and tried to portray an atmosphere of calm and confidence. Collectively, we have managed several patients similar to Hank before and successfully administered the prescribed 15 dosages of PEG asparaginase in accordance with the protocol. However, the initial anxiety, at the moment of truth, always caused time to stand still.

The infusion began and we could see the drug make its way through the IV tubing, enter the port-a-catheter, and slowly into the patient. Less than one minute later, after having received less than 5 ml of the infusion Hank's color turned blue, and he developed an erythematous red, papular rash on his trunk and back. He looked as if he had measles; an obvious allergic reaction.

"Stop! Stop immediately!"

Hank's blood pressure dropped; his cardiovascular system was under attack. Jane Stark, one of the oncology nurse practitioners, listened to his lungs with her stethoscope.

"He's wheezing. His heart rate is down to 50."

"Give him another dose of methylprednisolone and the epinephrine, a normal saline bolus and the oxygen."

Hank cried out," Mommy, mommy!"

He vomited, and now another concern was aspiration. Jane cleaned him quickly and suctioned his mouth removing the vomitus. Hank gagged and cried; he was choking.

Heather and Max were terrified. Within the three months their son had a craniotomy for a malignant brain tumor, was diagnosed with leukemia, and now his life was threatened by an allergic, full-blown anaphylactic reaction.

"Call a RAPID!"

A RAPID is a hospital-wide alert that a patient is unstable, in dire need of an immediate escalation in care. Its intent is to rapidly assess hospitalized patients with altered and changing vital signs, and intervene quickly to avoid potential disasters such as a cardiac arrest or respiratory failure that necessitate an upstaging of care and a transfer to an intensive care unit. At New York Presbyterian, Columbia University Medical Center there is a RAPID team for the Milstein Pavilion, the adult hospital, and one for the Morgan Stanley Children's Hospital. When Carin Schultz called the RAPID, it triggered a response by the pediatric team of critical care nurses, residents on the PICU rotation, and critical care fellows to respond urgently.

The concept of a RAPID is just that—it is intended to be instantaneous. However, our clinic is located in the Irving Pavilion, so to reach Hank, the RAPID team was required to depart the critical care unit on the ninth floor of the Morgan Stanley Children's Hospital, race down the stairs to the third floor, traverse the long hallway through the Presbyterian Hospital and the Harkness Pavilion, cross the pedestrian bridge over Fort Washington Avenue into the Milstein Hospital building, make a sharp left down the corridor and enter the Irving Pavilion on the fifth floor, race to the stairwell, ascend two flights to the seventh floor and then proceed to the back corner of the pediatric oncology outpatient unit.

I walk this route frequently. It is more than half a mile in distance and takes between 7 and 12 minutes depending on your pace. Thus, our pediatric oncology doctors and nurses were tasked with stabilizing Hank until the RAPID team arrived. In such emergency situations, my experience informs that the fellows and nurse practitioners are more adept and knowledgeable than the attendings. This was certainly the situation on this particular Tuesday afternoon. Laila Ratner, an exceptional, confident third-year fellow took charge of Hank's immediate management.

Laila ordered, "Jessica, Carin, start another peripheral IV, draw a set of electrolytes, and send them STAT. Run normal saline as fast as possible through the new line. Give another dose of epinephrine 0.01 milligrams IV. Jane, what are his vital signs now?"

"Blood pressure is 80/55, pulse, 60, pulse oxygen is 80; he is still wheezing, still blue."

I was an observer. My role was to take Hank's parents out of the room, away from the immediacy, the controlled chaos of their son's dire situation of circulatory collapse. I tried to keep calm and reassure them. Watching Hank struggle to breathe, with unstable vital signs, covered in a rash, his clothes soaked in his regurgitated breakfast of Cheerios and milk would be terrifying for any parent. But, being a physician, Heather understood every nuance of care, could not extricate herself from the bedside; she needed to watch every detail, to participate in the resuscitation though she knew that was not possible. I told them that we would get Hank through this episode of shock and awe. Heather's training informed that I was correct, but it did not diminish the fact that, first and foremost, she was a mother and her son was in trouble. Max, on the other hand, was frozen—a deer in the headlights.

The RAPID team finally arrived from the critical care unit, panting, out of breath. The team consisted of several residents, two critical care nurses, and Tamara Martone, the nurse manager for the children's hospital. The senior resident, Chris Rogers, was in charge. "What are the latest vital signs?"

Mary repeated the numbers.

"Let's move him to the PICU now. Call the unit and tell them we need an emergency bed and are transporting the patient now. How much steroids has he received?"

Jessica replied, "He's gotten methylprednisolone, 100 mg IV twice."

"Okay, give him another dose and get him ready to move. Also give another dose of Benadryl 15 mg IV. Call security to hold an elevator in this building and also a CHONY central elevator. Put the oxygen tank on the bed, keep the nasal cannula going at 3 liters of oxygen, get an ambu bag. Draw up another dose of epi and take it with us. Let's go!"

I had a lot of confidence in Chris Rogers. He was a third-year resident and would soon embark on a fellowship in pediatric cardiology at Boston Children's Hospital, one of the best training programs in the country. I have known Chris since he was a toddler; his parents Thomas and Nobuko Rogers, both physicians, had been our friends for many years and were our neighbors in Tenafly, New Jersey. I have also worked with Chris during his residency as an oncology attending on Tower 5; he is an excellent doctor.

The team released the brakes on the hospital bed and began to move Hank and all the medical paraphernalia—IV poles, monitors, oxygen—towards the elevator. Heather, Tom, and I trailed Hank and the team transporting him. Rather than wait for the elevators, Heather, Tom, and I raced for the stairs. We retraced the route that the RAPID team had traveled moments before. When we got to the children's hospital, there happened to be a North Building elevator available, we got in, pressed 9, and exited. I needed to use my ID card at the security card reader, and magically, it worked. We walked together to the 9 Central ICU and found Hank in Room 10. The critical care nurses and the team led by Chris Rogers and Roger Carroll, Director of the Division of Critical Care, were doing an initial assessment, connecting monitoring leads and making certain the port-catheter line and the peripheral line in Hank's right arm were all functioning and running well. His nurse, Shadra, reported and recorded his vital signs: "Heart rate 100; BP, 90/65; respiratory rate, 30; oxygen saturation, 95; temp, 99."

Looking over at Hank's parents I saw my relief reflected tenfold in their faces. His color improved, rash fading, vitals back to baseline, breathing comfortably, he fell asleep from the naroleptic effect of the Benadryl; he survived. Shadra removed his soiled Polo Ralph Lauren shirt and pants, placing them in a white plastic bag for safekeeping.

As Heather began to cry, Max said, "Thanks, Dr. Weiner. We thought we would lose him; that was terrifying, the most frightening ordeal we have ever experienced. No more asparaginase—promise."

He held his wife who spoke in a very soft voice, "Thank you."

"I understand; I was concerned."

The truth is that I had done very little during the emergency. The expert team of residents and nurses were extraordinary and unflappable. There is a good reason why the reputation of Columbia University Children's Health and Morgan Stanley Children's Hospital is the singular best place to be for care in the New York area.

"Thank God for that."

The Pandemic

Hank Held and Chaya Lefkowitz were adorable, engaging toddlers. Medically unique, they had wonderful families, who I got to know over the course of their treatment and care. They shared rare but different presentations of leukemia. It's a challenging prognosis for any family, however, once the shock of their diagnosis had settled and treatment was initiated, they both responded quite well.

Hank had short-cropped, light brown hair, sparkling blue eyes, and an athletic build for a three-year-old. He was always nattily dressed in Ralph Lauren polo shirts and sweaters, chinos, and tiny Nike sneakers. Invariably, he carried a Matchbox toy car and truck, and his lunchbox was filled with a peanut butter and jelly sandwich, potato chips, banana, and an Oreo cookie. On clinic days, he always had an iPad to watch *Thomas the Tank Engine*, *PAW Patrol*, or *Toy Story* videos.

As if being diagnosed with two simultaneous, synchronous cancers, a brain tumor, and acute lymphoblastic leukemia were not enough, Hank almost died secondary to a severe anaphylactic reaction to PEG asparaginase. Despite this trauma, he subsequently settled in and had a seamless, uneventful course. His leukemia remained in a continuous, complete remission for three years, and the routine MRIs of his brain every three to six months to monitor the status of the previously resected brain tumor were excellent, displaying no evidence of re-emergence.

Hank's protocol, a Children's Oncology Group standard risk regimen, required monthly clinic visits for blood work and intravenous vincristine. More often than not, he was accompanied by his father, Max, who was between jobs. Max was a big guy, almost 6-feet, 5-inches, affable, and regardless of the season wore Allbirds, an extremely comfortable shoe made in New Zealand, in either navy blue or tan. Until recently, Max had worked for the Hunt brothers, wealthy Texas oil barons, managing their diversified real estate assets but had left after a falling out with them regarding investment strategy and compensation. His severance sufficient to afford him time to investigate new opportunities, he was in no rush to start anew, and most assuredly wanted to be his own boss and make his own investment decisions. He enjoyed this newfound time with his son; they both relished coming to clinic, and quite frankly, I welcomed my time with the Held boys.

Hank's mother, Heather Pace, feeling confident in Luke's recovery, returned to work. She relinquished her position as a special fertility fellow at Mt. Sinai—it was an impossible time commitment—and took a faculty position at Yale New Haven in general obstetrics. However, Yale was onerous as well, time wise, and she was hired by West Med, a large multi-specialty group in Westchester near the family home in Rye. Her new position seemed perfect in every respect. Heather accompanied Hank and Max every three months, the beginning of a new 84-day chemotherapy cycle, and the day of a scheduled lumbar puncture performed in the ENDO suite under conscious sedation—a big day.

I introduced Max and Heather to the Hope & Heroes Children's Fund, knowing that they were the type of family who would be needed to sustain the charity in the future if it was to succeed—young, affluent, with school-age children, committed to their community, and passionate about helping children like their son.

Two members of our board, Sam Queen and Mickey Bowen, invited me and Max to play golf at Fenway Country Club; and he joined our foursome of Dean Lee Sterngold, Herb Roberts, and myself at our golf outing at Wing Foot. Max was a good player with an 8–9 handicap, but what was most impressive was that, with his size, strength, and new Callaway Rogue driver, he hit the golf ball more than 300 yards off the tee. He and Heather attended our annual dinner at Chelsea Piers, where I introduced them to Lauren and Eli; amazingly, they were contemporaries but seemed more mature somehow. Having a child with cancer tends to do that to young couples.

———————

Although we were not able to enroll Chaya on the Dana-Farber leukemia protocol because she had received intensive prior steroids to treat the immune system dysregulation. Our leukemia team, Carol Justice, Tiki Tanaka, and I, decided to follow the treatment plan, adhering to high-risk protocol, adding Doxorubicin and high-dose methotrexate as intensification. It was the correct decision. Chaya was a cherubic little doll, hairless from the chemotherapy, cushingoid cheeks from the Decadron, an oversized personality for her two and a half years of age, and the vocabulary of a much older child.

Always polite, she would greet me when I entered her room: "Good morning, Dr. Weiner! How are you today?"

"I'm fine today, Chaya. How are you?"

"I'm good. Mommy brought me to clinic; I have a cheese sandwich for lunch today."

Chaya tolerated treatment extremely well. The only wrinkle was a little gastrointestinal upset, mild pancreatitis caused by the PEG asparaginase. Otherwise, she uneventfully entered a complete remission, had a low MRD (minimal residual disease), and continues to do well to this day.

One day in early March 2020, Jill Duncan, one of the leukemia team nurse practitioners, received a call at the clinic from Mrs. Lefkowitz informing us that Mr. Lefkowitz was ill. He had a high fever, a cough, and generally felt lousy. His primary doctor thought it was the flu, despite his having had a flu shot, and prescribed Tamiflu, an anti-influenza treatment. Neither Chaya nor anyone else at home was ill, at least not yet, and she indicated that she would not be able to bring Chaya for her regular appointment and asked to postpone the visit for a week.

Mr. Lefkowitz, a Talmudic scholar and teacher, taught a class at a *yeshiva* in New Rochelle, New York, a small suburban city just north of Manhattan and the Bronx. Recent news from New Rochelle reported that the Coronavirus—a novel respiratory infection that seemingly had begun in Wuhan, China, but was quickly sweeping the globe—was present in the community and spreading rapidly. Could Mr. Lefkowitz have this deadly virus? Could the virus be similar to SARS or H1N1? One thing was certain, he was sick; not hospital-requiring sick, but bedridden at home and sick for four days. By the end of the week, Mr. Lefkowitz's health had improved, but his wife was ill with the same symptoms: high fever, cough, sore throat, body aches and pains. Chaya and her two brothers and sister seemed to all contract the virus as well but had only mild symptoms, displaying a very low-grade fever for a day or two.

By March, the Coronavirus (COVID-19) was multiplying rapidly in Europe, with the Tuscany region of northern Italy and Spain particularly hard hit. The number of cases soon reached the tens of thousands, and before long, New York City had become the epicenter of the virus, with thousands dying as the city, state, and country worked desperately to contain the virus' spread with inadequate equipment and treatments. Practically overnight, New York Presbyterian and the other city hospitals were overwhelmed, with doctors fashioning makeshift coverings out of garbage bags as ill New Yorkers desperately waited and died in hospital hallways.

The Centers for Disease Control (CDC) and the New York State Department of Health (NYDOH) reported that men over 65 years of age with preexisting medical conditions were at a particularly increased risk of severe disease and death. I checked all three boxes. I sent instant messages to Kim Kindle, my internist; Debra Lawrence, my oncologist; and Maxine Morris, a friend and virologist, and asked their opinions regarding work at the hospital. The message was clear—stay at home, you're at high risk, isolate. I notified Daniel Hito, the newly appointed division director, and Sharon Malamud, the division administrator, that I would be working remotely and suspending patient contact and would, therefore, not be available for my assigned Tuesday clinic sessions until there was greater clarity about COVID-19, risks of infection, and an official policy from New York Presbyterian and Columbia University Irving Medical Center. I also forwarded the emails I had received from my doctors and Maxine Morris. The new hospital and university directives were that there was no immediate policy. The entire institution was caught off guard and unprepared; chaos prevailed.

The next week was terrifying. Chaya, still febrile, had to be seen, blood counts had to be obtained, and blood cultures drawn. On Tuesday, during a routine clinic visit, we learned that the father of Jacki Ramirez Campo, a three-year-old leukemia patient, had been admitted to the intensive care unit at Harlem Hospital in dire condition and was now on a ventilator. Chaya and Jacki had both clearly been exposed to COVID-19 through their fathers. A patient with sickle-cell anemia, Shaquille Edwards, arrived on Wednesday with fever, gastrointestinal symptoms, and a severe headache—he too had apparently contracted the virus. There could be no doubt that COVID-19 was in our midst.

Friday evening, Herb Roberts called. I knew that whatever he needed, it must have been of great importance as it was *Shabbos* and he rarely made phone calls from sundown Friday through Saturday evening. Herb told me his daughter, Shari, an oncology nurse on Irving-7, was sick with a high fever, cough, and shortness of breath—she was on her way to the emergency room. He asked me to make a few calls to expedite her visit. I notified Dean Sterngold and Evan Greene, who in turn called the emergency room so the triage nurse was expecting her. Fortunately, Shari's respiratory capacity was acceptable with oxygen saturation above 90 percent. However, she spent the next 10 days isolated from her husband, children, and family.

Luci Drakos called Sunday night; her husband, Constantine, Head of Child and Adolescent Neuro-Oncology, a personal friend and a terrific doctor, couldn't breathe, had an unrelenting cough, and a fever of 103 degrees. "Michael, I'm worried."

I asked her to put Constantine on the phone.

"I'll try."

He could barely talk or breathe between coughs. Calmly, I suggested to Luci that she find someone to care for her daughters and take her husband to the ER. She told me that her father was visiting from London, no worries about the girls. I messaged the Dean and Evan and once again they worked their magic. Thankfully, Constantine did not need admission to the hospital, but he remained quite ill for two weeks before he began slowly to recover. Luci became ill with the Coronavirus as well but had an abbreviated and less severe course of illness.

My wife, Alicia, and I adore Constantine and Luci. Constantine was Greek; Luci, a dentist with a particular interest in treating oral manifestations of cancer patients, is Iranian. An elegant couple, they met in London. We were fortunate to recruit Constantine to Columbia. His clinical intellect, patient skills, and mentorship of the fellows was extraordinary; he possessed unteachable leadership qualities. He also proved to be a capable fundraiser and secured more than $2 million from the Frost and Dillon Foundations to support his novel drug delivery research initiative in children with diffuse pontine glioma—an uncurbable type of brain tumor. Now, by his own admission, he was more ill than ever before.

Arush Krishana and Meredith Lin from the stem cell transplant team and hematology, respectively, also contracted the virus, their symptoms mild and illnesses relatively short.

As the influenza pandemic of 1918 shaped a long-ago era, so too the Coronavirus pandemic of 2020 has defined lives at Columbia and the Morgan Stanley Children's Hospital of New York Presbyterian. The impact was sudden, tragic, acute, and not unlike the terrorist attack on the World Trade

Center on September 11, 2001; our city became the country's medical center ground zero.

The number of patients with COVID-19 escalated rapidly from the first hospitalization in February, to tens of cases, to hundreds, to thousands of patients in a matter of days. The first department to experience this sudden, dramatic influx was the emergency room. Even under the best of circumstances the ER is hectic, but this situation was different as patients doubled-up in rooms, stretchers languished in the halls, and teams roamed the hospital seeking equipment and monitors. The staff, nurses, and doctors were multitasking, and the ER in March 2020 was akin to a war zone field hospital. The ever-increasing number of sick patients—white, black, and brown, young and old alike—stressed the system beyond comprehension. Walk-in patients lined up to be triaged, and the EMT service was swamped 24 hours a day, 7 days a week, bringing patients to Columbia University Irving Medical Center (CUIMC), coughing and unable to breathe. Many were placed on respirators before they even had vital signs obtained.

The existing medical and surgical intensive care units in the Milstein Hospital building were inadequate to manage the caseload. Additional capacity was needed. New York Presbyterian quickly came together to convert the operating rooms on the 4th floor, the ENDO-Bronchoscopy procedure rooms on the 11th floor of the Irving Pavilion, the cardiac catheterization suites, and the pediatric critical care beds in the Morgan Stanley Children's Hospital (CHONY) into adult ICU beds. Ventilators were in short supply, and at times, two patients shared a single respirator as urgent decisions had to be made.

In the midst of the bedlam, Max Held sent me an email to ask my opinion about the family travelling to Naples, Florida, to visit Heather's parents. I inquired as to how they would be travelling.

"JetBlue."

I told Max that despite a paucity of scientific data it seemed unsafe to travel by commercial airlines. "I honestly believe it safer not to make the trip; stay home, isolate, don't take any chances. Florida will always be there."

He countered that everyone was healthy and the kids were looking forward to spending time with the grandparents. Max, Heather, Hank, Brittany, and six-month-old Casey made the trip, had a great time swimming in the pool, and playing on the beach bathed by warm Gulf of Mexico water. The Held family returned to New York by private jet, but shortly thereafter, Hank, Max, and Brittany became ill with the Coronavirus. Max and Brittany had mild illness, low-grade fever, sore throat and Brittany had gastrointestinal symptoms and pain. But Hank developed higher fever that necessitated a visit to the hospital for blood counts, cultures and two days of ceftriaxone; fortunately, he recovered uneventfully, but we all agreed that the risk of the trip had been too great—lesson learned.

Hospital and university leadership including Michael Winters and Peg Edwards, Chief Executive Officer and Executive Vice President of New York Presbyterian, respectively, as well as Dean Sterngold and George Childs, President of Columbia Doctors, were the field marshals and generals, rallying their troops of doctors, nurses, respiratory therapists, administrators, dietary staff, housekeeping, and maintenance staff. Everyone was needed; everyone was considered mission critical—the definition of "essential workers". The institution's resources were stretched beyond the breaking point. The war against COVID-19 was being waged without sufficient ammunition as the Coronavirus, the invisible foe, gained an upper hand. It was as if the battle was being waged in the trenches of World War I, the enemy employing missiles and stealth bombers.

Stories from Italy, a country whose healthcare system was totally overrun by the COVID-19 pandemic, began to circulate about doctors who were "God-playing"—prioritizing those with the highest chances of survival, meaning the young and the healthy over those older than 65 years of age or with pre-existing medical conditions. They strongly advised against allocating precious resources, like ventilators and beds, on the traditional basis of first-come, first-served, which would reduce the number of lives a hospital could save. Care was rationed and those with the highest likelihood of survival were chosen, rather than expend precious resources, medication, respirators, and dialysis machines on patients deemed less likely to survive. Naturally, we began to question whether this unspeakable, apocalyptic reality could come to New York Presbyterian. The answer was a resounding no.

Columbia and NYP would not under any circumstances ration care, even if approaching maximum capacity limits. The hospital mandated that high-intensity, mostly successful care must be delivered as long as the other resources, including healthcare workers that support complex care delivery, did not exceed capacity. Being forced to make choices regarding life and death is not part of our institutional DNA.

As March evolved into April, the nightmare worsened. It was apparent that the personal protective equipment (PPE) needed to protect healthcare workers on the front line was an increasingly limited resource. N95 respirator masks, face shields, and gowns needed to safeguard against droplet spread of the virus were scarce commodities. I learned that prior to the pandemic, throughout the NYP system hospitals, approximately 4,000 non-N95 masks were used each day; now with the Coronavirus upon us, the usage exceeded 70,000 per day. Employees were administered one non-N95 mask, asked to protect it, guard it, and place in a paper bag at the end of their shift to be used another day. The mask was as valuable as gold.

Doctors, nurses, and staff were angry. They felt vulnerable and compromised as the systems around them failed and the institutions meant to protect them as well as their patients fell short. But there was no one to blame; the situation was unprecedented. No amount of preparation could have prevented the onslaught healthcare workers and other first responders dealt with every minute of every hour of every day.

Some became sick, isolated, and quarantined. A few actually died. Maxoaki Miko, Chief of the Solid Organ Transplant Program and an internationally renowned surgeon, became ill and spent three weeks on a respirator in the

ICU. Others yielded to the immense pressure, and one emergency room physician, unable to manage the mounting tension and stressful demands of work, committed suicide.

The NYP system and our hospital, as well as other New York City institutions, was losing the battle. At CUIMC, there were 1,000 patients infected with the virus and 600 on ventilators, with PPE in short and dwindling supply. A tent was erected outside the emergency room on 168th Street to triage patients; fever clinics were opened; and a 200-bed field hospital was built by the National Guard Army Corp of Engineers at Baker Field, Columbia University's athletic stadium on 218th Street, adjacent to the Allen Pavilion. The structure accommodated overflow cases not needing an ICU in the Milstein building.

Drs. Miller and Edwards gave daily updates on the numbers of hospitalized patients as well as rapidly evolving policy guidelines for healthcare workers, the status of PPE, and the availability of PCR nasal swab testing. Collaborating with Dean Sterngold and George Childs, elective surgery and procedures were suspended. Only urgent medical care was rendered on site—patients with impending emergencies, myocardial infections, stroke, and adults and children with cancer were admitted and treated—all others were denied access into the hospital buildings. Routine visits were converted to telemedicine. The entire research enterprise at Columbia, one of the great academic centers in the world, except for COVID-19 related investigations deemed critical, was temporarily suspended.

Physician activities for the majority of doctors on the faculty came to a grinding halt. Internists, Emergency Department doctors, and intensivists were crushed under the weight of responsibilities levied upon them; they worked with little rest and often for multiple days without time off. The cry for help was heard loud and clear; the solution, re-deployment. Adaptability, resolve, and self-sacrifice were the only tools to fight back.

The Weill Cornell east side campus of NYP experienced a similar surge in COVID-19 cases. To accommodate adult patients, the inpatient unit at the Komansky Children's Center closed and all pediatric patients requiring hospital admission were transferred and accepted at Columbia, MSCHONY. The intensive care units in the Morgan Stanley Children's Hospital terminated care to children and ramped up to accommodate critical adult patients. Pediatricians, residents, fellows, pediatric nurse practitioners, and physician assistants helped with the case load, managing 40- to 50-year-old patients. Roger Carroll told me that, despite the obvious personal risk, it was energizing to be in the middle of the fight; he and his colleagues and staff were thrilled to work and contribute.

Stories abound about the courage and inspiration of healthcare workers. New heroes praised and glorified for their service on the front line, rightfully lauded as New York's finest and bravest, these doctors, nurses, therapists, and hospital employees, who risked their lives to go above and beyond their call of duty, helped New York and America as a whole to put an end to the spread. Each evening at 7, New Yorkers across the five boroughs cheered and clapped for their new heroes.

I experienced significant internal conflict. Doctors were needed, and around me, colleagues were making the difficult decision to continue working and caring for children with cancer—patients and families needed them. I was safely sheltered at our home in Salisbury, Connecticut, with Alicia, our son Eli, his wife, Carolyn, and two dogs, Clementine and Molly. I was racked with guilt, tormented really, and each day I questioned whether I should be in clinic, seeing kids, doing lumbar punctures and bone marrows, and doing my share. I even contemplated re-deployment to a COVID-19 unit. However, my instincts for survival and risk avoidance superseded any compunction about returning to the hospital. I remained isolated at home, working remotely. I was incredibly busy working on any number of projects for the division and in my role as vice chair of external affairs for the department of pediatrics. We launched email newsletters and public service video interviews and webinars, yet I continued to be conflicted. I needed to do more.

All conferences across the enterprise, hospital, and university were converted to virtual video via Zoom and Webex. I participated in every update, meeting, teaching round, and discussion. Tower 5, the inpatient oncology floor, remained open and there were three or four COVID-19 positive patients on the unit at all times. Only patients who required scheduled chemotherapy and procedures were permitted in the clinic. Routine patient visits, off-therapy children, and survivor wellness patients were postponed or converted to telemedicine visits. The pediatric oncology staff was reduced significantly to one attending physician and one nurse practitioner—no ambulatory fellows. All worked from home, but still, I felt guilty and conflicted.

There was one thing that I knew that I could do and do well—raise money to help others. I worked with Brooks Calub, Director of Hyundai Hope on Wheels, to secure a $200,000 gift to support the first clinic in the country dedicated to the care of infants born to Coronavirus-infected and -ill mothers. I worked with Sam and Cecile Queen, friends and Hope & Heroes board members, who wanted to do something to help healthcare workers at the hospital. The Queens donated $150,000 and challenged their friends and business associates to match their donation. Their efforts raised $327,000. Karl Washington, Executive Director of the Hope & Heroes Children's Cancer Fund, at my suggestion, created a special account, the Hope & Heroes COVID-19 Fund, to be gifted to the Department of Pediatrics. Randy Willis, Chief Financial Officer of the Department, identified that one of the most stressful aspects for pediatric learners, residents, and fellows was traveling to the hospital and home again on public transportation. The city was in lockdown; subways and buses were dangerous, unclean, and infrequently operated. Randy created a Lyft account and administered a code number to each caregiver in order to permit their safe travel anytime, day or night. In addition, funds from the account provided free meals to employees while in the hospital and personal financial assistance to children with cancer and their families for whatever they needed.

I volunteered to work for New York Presbyterian's Work Force Health and Safety (WHS), an employee hotline created to provide guidance and answer Coronavirus related questions. NYP has eight hospitals, geographically situated from Queens to Brooklyn to lower Manhattan to Westchester, and more than 50,000 racially, ethnically, and socio-economically diverse employees, all terrified, vulnerable, and/or sick. I worked three shifts per week—Sunday, Wednesday, and Friday mornings from 6 to 10—from mid-March to the end of May. I found calm during these early morning shifts; they afforded me some measure of peace, knowing that I was doing what I could to contribute without unnecessarily jeopardizing my own life. Initially, the calls came fast and furious, all horrific.

I vividly remember a call from a respiratory therapist at NYP Queens who told me that her mother became ill with fever, cough, and had difficulty breathing. She had gone to her mother's apartment in the Bronx, called 911, and waited four hours for the ambulance that took her mother to Jacobi, a municipal hospital, where her mother died several hours later, alone. Now she was sick. She cried to me, "Please don't let me die."

I vividly remember a call from a medical resident at Weill Cornell, assigned to work in the emergency department, who lived by herself in Greenwich Village. She was continuously and constantly exposed to scores of patients with COVID-19 and had contracted the disease. Now sick, her cough was so severe that she could barely speak. She tried calling 911 but to no avail. I suggested she call a friend or neighbor and ask them to take her to the ED; I gave her my name and mobile number and asked her to call when she arrived at Cornell. Three hours later, she called, on oxygen, feeling better, and being cared for by her friends and colleagues. She called again three weeks later to tell me that she had completely recovered and was back at work: "Thank you."

Work Force Health and Safety maintained an Excel spreadsheet to record and document each call. In early April, during the height of the caseload surge in New York City, there were thousands of employee names on the list, with 10 percent of the NYP workforce out of work, at home, on isolation, or sick with Coronavirus. In May, although the volume of calls remained high, the questions and issues changed. The hospital was less dangerous, employees had appropriate personal protective equipment, the lockdown rigidly enforced by Mayor de Blasio and Governor Cuomo, reduced the city and statewide caseload, and beds and ventilators were more readily available. Employees called the hotline for return to work clearance or to schedule a COVID-19 PCR nasal swab test or a serological antibody test. NYP now had the capacity to test all employees, and every patient that entered any building at Columbia University Irving Medical Center was screened at entry and mandated to wear a mask and social distance six feet apart.

On June 1st, with great trepidation, I decided to return to work. I was prepared to take all necessary precautions to be safe and keep Alicia and my family safe and infection-free. I would wear a scrub suit, masks, eye shield, gown, and N95 respirator mask. I would remain in my office with the door closed and only venture out when absolutely necessary to see a patient. Throughout the day, I would use Purell often. I was prepared to have lunch at my desk and continue all conferences and meetings via Zoom. At the end of the day, I would remove the PPE, change back into street clothes in my office, toss the scrubs in the soiled clothing hamper, quietly take the back stairs, and exit the building out to 165th Street to the parking lot, get in my teal blue BMW 330i, and drive home to Ardsley. At home, I would immediately doff my clothes in the hallway bathroom, place them in the washing machine, and take a long, hot shower.

On the positive side, Hank Held and Chaya Lefkowitz were both well after overcoming their Coronavirus infections; I was excited to see them both.

Evan Greene, Chair of Pediatrics, led his department of 300 faculty, 150 learners, residents and fellows, and a staff in the hundreds. He was inspirational, supportive, calm, and informative; he recognized the needs of his team members, young and old, as great leaders do. Dr. Greene led from the front, set an example of high standards, and espoused unremitting gratitude and thanks. Working with Randy Willis, Chief Financial Officer of the department, and Lara Castinova, Vice Chair for Education, they developed POWER, an exhaustive resource of information and psycho-emotional help for the staff. The department innovated in numerous ways, creating the Newborn COVID-19 center and the dedicated COVID-19 Fund which provided Lyft rides for physicians, residents and staff, enabling them to travel to and from the hospital, and offered meals and on-campus housing if needed. The department created a research collaborative to study, share, and publish articles about this new disease, the novel COVID-19.

The story is far from complete; the pandemic continues to rage across the country, with greater than 5 million cases diagnosed and 175,000 deaths. The future is uncertain.

Epilogue

As I conclude these pages, the future of our country feels tenuous as the United States sits poised on a precipice. We are struggling with the fallout of so many neglected crises, from containing the Coronavirus pandemic, to effectively dealing with climate change, to addressing our country's long, insidious, and vile history of racial inequity. It is well beyond the scope of this book to offer adequate solutions regarding these important issues. It is not that I lack passion or that I am apolitical, but rather that I am not the right person with the right expertise to address these complex challenges. Much of our current landscape seems to me to be the result of men with power overreaching and overestimating the breadth of their own understanding, and I do not intend to do that in these pages. What I did set out to do, and what I hope I've accomplished, is to relate with sincerity, heart, and some humor my experiences with cancer, viewed from every angle; from caregiver to doctor to parent and survivor.

Lauren remains well. She religiously takes thyroid replacement therapy, remains health- and wellness-conscious, is married, and has two beautiful children—a son and daughter.

I am well also. The follicular lymphoma continues to be quiescent, in complete remission. With each day, each week, each month without relapse, the odds of cure increase. Or do they? Despite the fact that my physical exam, PET/CT scans, and blood work remain normal, at each follow-up, Dr. Lawrence reminds me that there are no cures. Patients don't die from follicular lymphoma; they die with follicular lymphoma. She continues to say that it is only a matter of time until recurrence, relapse, and assuredly chemotherapy, probably Bendamustine. As Lauren asked on numerous occasions, "What choice do I have?"

I am also dealing with the thyroid nodule, now increased in size to 9 mm from 6 mm. Dr. Tom James told me that at 10 mm, a biopsy is warranted and that he believes the lesion is probably a slow-growing papillary thyroid cancer. There's nothing to do at this juncture but to wait and be patient. I recognize what lies ahead—thyroidectomy, radioactive iodine . . . "What choice do I have?"

The changing landscape of healthcare precipitated by COVID-19 and a shift in our nation's awareness of systemic racism and equality has altered my work at Columbia, New York Presbyterian. It is different. The pandemic has forced many to re-evaluate careers and retirement. Such decisions are difficult in the best of circumstances and are not unique to medicine. However, in the wake of the ongoing pandemic, certainly medicine has its unique challenges. Professionals and employees of large companies in virtually any industry struggle to find that right moment to "hang up the proverbial spikes," at the top of one's game while still relevant and not on the decline.

I recognize that I am no longer the future of our division of oncology. Daniel Hito, one of the first physicians I recruited 24 years ago, is the new division director. I have always had high regard for Daniel. He is a good person and a good doctor, but his path to effective leadership is long. He must learn to be decisive, to support his faculty, and to curtail fomenting dissension that adversely affects morale. Our relationship remains excellent. While I have offered to provide insight and be a sounding board, and though we do talk periodically, he has chosen to rely on others as his inner sanctum of advisors. I have learned to accept this changing role.

James Bergen, the department chair who hired me, is long gone from the hospital, as is Don Colbert. James had a recent devastating stroke that left him cognitively intact but unable to speak. His rehabilitation is rigorous, his progress slow. Don Colbert was appointed Vice Dean for Global Initiatives, a well-suited position for him to pursue his interests in food insecurity and vaccination programs in Africa. He has traveled to more than 100 countries around the globe and always seems to have his bags packed. Unfortunately, the pandemic has significantly curtailed his scientific and humanitarian expeditions.

The present chair of the department of pediatrics, Evan Greene, is very much in control. In less than two years he has reshaped the department, instituting numerous changes in leadership, division directorship, new programs, creating his team comprised of his contemporaries, mid-career, intelligent, hard-working.

Although I remain a vice chair of the department and member of the executive committee, my role has diminished. Whereas I had played an important role in development and outreach, these responsibilities have now been assumed by others. I coined the phrase "Columbia Children's Health" and created the Children's Board at Columbia with Lara Bendix, VP for Development, during Don Colbert's time as chair. When Lara departed the institution, my role with the board diminished.

Evan wants to conduct his own philanthropic efforts—his call.

I am convinced that Evan Greene's vision to be one of the best children's hospitals in the country in clinical care, research, and education will be realized. He has succeeded in every endeavor he has previously undertaken; he has charisma, extraordinary intelligence, and natural leadership qualities.

All of this change requires a tremendous adjustment, not only in outlook, attitude, and day-to-day. Remaining useful, relevant, of value—this looks different now than it once did. I struggled to find my niche and to understand what I could add to the division and to the department that would allow me to work and remain employed. I continue to see patients with leukemia and lymphoma, and patient care remains joyful and fulfilling. I continue to participate in conferences and oncology rounds. I continue to teach and mentor hematology-oncology fellows. I continue to oversee and participate in the operation of the Hope & Heroes Children's Cancer

Fund—the scope of this responsibility alone could be a full-time occupation. Truth be known, Hope & Heroes provides and supports more than 40 percent of the division's operating budget. I embody the foundation. Daniel Hito understands that significance, as do Evan Greene and Dean Sterngold.

An interesting piece of this metamorphosis: I have taken on the responsibility of marketing and branding for the department. To tell its story, I work with Liz Gump and Group Gordon, a public relations firm, and together, we have created *The Check-Up*, a monthly internal newsletter and our first ever annual report for the department, with webinars, email newsletters, brochures, social media postings, and public service announcements. I am writing the history of the Babies Hospital, the first children's hospital in New York and second oldest in the United States, in order to keep its history alive. I am also editor of the second edition of *Secrets of Pediatric Hematology-Oncology*, a textbook soon to be published.

I am fortunate that my health is good, my work is fulfilling, and my relevance and value are secure. I believe that I will be able to work for as long as I desire, on my terms—a very good thing.

Alicia and I enjoy time at our home in Salisbury, Connecticut. We have a full, rich, active life, which we share with a number of close, dear friends, many of whom we have known for decades. Recently, we had to upgrade the sprinkler system and drip hoses for Alicia's raised bed vegetable garden and better coverage for the lawn. The owner/salesperson from Northeast Irrigation came to our home on Ravine Ridge, introduced himself, and handed me his business card, introducing himself as Eric Logalbo.

"Eric, are you related to the Logalbo family in northern New Jersey? Do you know Carlie and her mother, Melanie?"

"Carlie is my younger sister, and Melanie my mom."

"Eric, I'm Dr. Weiner, Michael Weiner. I took care of your sister decades ago when she was ill with myelogenous leukemia."

Eric and I recalled the miracle, Melanie's visit to pray with Cardinal Cooke, Carlie's dream, her survival, and cure. Eric told me that Carlie, now 50, has three children and lives in Saddle River, New Jersey. What better way to end this story than to contemplate one of the most memorable and important events of my life.

Acknowledgements

The number of people to thank for making this book possible is long, and without the support and contribution of each and every one of them this book would not have been possible. Please recall that all the names except my own have been changed to protect privacy. The names of patients, parents, and families are fictitious, my colleagues including my personal doctors and my family, fabricated.

The stories I have chosen to tell have been selected from thousands of patients I have had the privilege of caring for in my 40-year career, each unique, powerful, and a learning experience. But the seven patients I recount in *Living Cancer* are those that had great impact upon me personally; some heart-wrenching that ended with the tragic death of a precious child despite our best collective medical expertise and effort. Others resulted in triumph, cancer vanquished, a life saved and family restored. However, regardless of the outcome, each patient experience, every family relationship, shaped and molded my personality and the person I am today.

Reflecting upon the hundreds of patients whose lives have been spared, perhaps in some small measure secondary to my guidance, brings me great joy. I try to remain in contact with as many as possible; among their ranks are doctors, lawyers, entrepreneurs, bankers, nurses, teachers, the career choices are endless. But, most importantly, many are married, have their own children, are mothers and fathers. Can one imagine the extraordinary bliss I feel meeting for the first time a new baby of a former patient? The proud surrogate grandfather.

I have special gratitude for Bill Oliver's parents, Anne and Steven. Anne's diary and the countless hours we spoke about her son are cherished memories and I continue to be crestfallen whenever I think about Bill and what might have been. I periodically see Anne and Steve at Hope & Heroes events and slowly detect that they are allowing their lives to proceed in a new normal. Your loss is immeasurable and we grieve for you every day.

I continue to be in awe of Frank and Madeline Nieman. Their strength and courage after the loss of their son, Mark Alan, is an example about how out of tragedy one may change the world and make it a better place. In their quest to understand Mark's illness, an unknown immunodeficiency disorder, they have enhanced scientific understanding of diseases of the immune system that has directly benefited children everywhere. Thank you, Frank and Madeline, for all that you do—remarkable, simply remarkable.

I have special thanks to Ellen Gomory, a young New Yorker now living in Birmingham, Alabama. I know Ellen by email and telephone only. We have never met in person, not for lack of trying, but the SARS-CoV-2 pandemic has made travel impossible. Ellen worked patiently with me, encouraged me, and guided the transformation of my writing. She allowed *Living Cancer* to be written.

My colleagues, attending physicians, fellows, nurse practitioners, nurses, social workers, administrative staff, and research coordinators have all made my years at Columbia University Irving Medical Center beyond great and pleasurable. To the three chairmen of the department of pediatrics that I served, thank you for your support and guidance. Together, each in your own manner and style worked with me to build a nationally recognized child and adolescent cancer program. To the three deans of the College of Physicians and Surgeons of Columbia University, and three executive directors of the New York Presbyterian Morgan Stanley Children's Hospital, thank you for your vision and creating an environment conducive to excellence inpatient care.

To my personal physicians, internist, surgeon, oncologists, and radiotherapist, thank you for your expertise and knowledge, but most importantly for being my partners on my personal cancer journey. You all have my deep gratitude.

I want to recognize and thank my daughter Lauren's physicians, surgeon, thyroid specialist, oncologist, and my friend Bruce Barry, her gynecologist, who tragically died in a bike accident.

Thank you, Atlantic Publishing, for giving me the opportunity to write and publish *Living Cancer*. Thank you, Kate Cline and Jesse Ranew for your editorial skill and responsiveness. Your professionalism and advice has been greatly appreciated.

Thank you Michael Gordon and Andrew Jarrell of Group Gordon, a public relations firm extraordinaire, for their advice and assistance in marketing my book.

Lastly, and most importantly I must thank my wife and family. My wife of 42 years for her constant, perpetual, love and admiration. Her encouragement, advice, and tolerance were instrumental in allowing me to complete *Living Cancer*. Thank you to my beautiful daughter for not only being the young woman she is today, married with two children, a boy and girl, an accomplished real estate asset manager at a major bank, but also allowing me to tell her story.

To my son, you are an inspiration and I always welcome your off-handed comments, you are awesome.

9 781620 237601